The Alternative Pregnanc Handbook

D1461721

For Iman and Shazia

TJ

For Steve, Coco and Bella

KE

The Alternative Pregnancy Handbook

DR TANVIR JAMIL AND KAREN EVENNETT

PIATKUS

Disclaimer: The contents of this book are for information only and are intended to assist
readers in identifying symptoms and conditions they may be experiencing. The book is not
intended to be a substitute for taking proper medical advice and should not be relied upon in
this way. Always consult a qualified doctor or health practitioner. The authors and the
publisher cannot accept responsibility for illness arising out of the failure to seek proper
medical advice.

Copyright © 2000 by
Tanvir Jamil and Karen Evennett
Published in the UK in 2000 by
Judy Piatkus (Publishers) Limited
5 Windmill Street
London W1T 2JA
e-mail: info@piatkus.co.uk

ISBN 0 7499 2117 X

Page design by Jerry Goldie
Edited by Carol Franklin

Data manipulation by Wyvern 21, Bristol

Printed and bound in Great Britain by
Butler & Tanner Ltd, Frome

CONTENTS

HOW TO USE THIS BOOK

Even if you have never previously taken an interest in complementary medicine, your pregnancy may seem like the ideal time to start.

Why? Because, on the whole, complementary medicine is safe – and as well as helping you solve the various problems (most of them minor, I hope!) which arise during the next year, it will enhance your general health and well-being.

I know from experience, while I was expecting my two daughters Coco and Bella, that many of the conventional over-the-counter treatments I would normally use without thinking, were not recommended during pregnancy. I found this frustrating, but didn't know of any reliable alternatives.

That is where this book comes in. It gives you the option of treating yourself using the safest natural remedies available – while also discussing recommended orthodox treatments. Homoeopathic remedies and many essential oils and herbal medicines are entirely safe to use in pregnancy – but should not be used carelessly. We aim to provide you with the practical information you need about safety issues, doses and when you should and shouldn't use different treatments.

Part One is a handy guide to conception, pregnancy and birth and what to do if you have a problem and want to know how best to treat it. We've then added a section on common childhood health problems that aims to help you in the first few months of your new baby's life. The final part of this book explains each of the complementary therapies and gives you all the facts about individual remedies to provide you with the background information you need.

Happy reading!

Karen Evennett
September 2000

INTRODUCTION

Welcome to this book. I often think that pregnancy is rather like watching a swan. On the surface there is beauty and grace whereas under the water there is a frantic effort to keep everything going just right. It's the same in pregnancy – you look beautiful and 'blooming' but underneath that healthy looking exterior your body is working flat out to keep you and your baby in prime condition. Your hormones are going up and down, your muscles and ligaments are being stretched, your body is storing up lots of fluid and your heart is working overtime.

Most of the time you will feel healthy and fine but sometimes all these changes can make you feel pretty rotten – we all know about early morning sickness, cravings and back pain but there are lots of other 'little' problems too. Your doctor can't do much about most of these conditions except prescribe the occasional drug and say that you will feel better once the baby is born.

Understandably most pregnant women are becoming more reluctant to take drugs and are increasingly turning towards complementary medicine as a way of helping some of the 'side-effects' of pregnancy. The other great advantage of these therapies is that you don't just have to use them if you have a problem. Therapies, such as meditation, yoga and the Alexander technique *keep* you healthy and relaxed and can stop certain problems from occurring in the first place. It's refreshing to be able to exert some control over what happens to you in pregnancy rather than just putting up with the difficulties.

Many women in my practice ask me if complementary medicines are safe in pregnancy. This is a very good question and safety has been the main consideration when writing this book. Complementary medicines are just like any other type of medical treatment and need to be given the same respect as conventional medicines. There are certain remedies that you cannot take during pregnancy, such as herbs and aromatherapy oils, and these have been listed in the various chapters. All the self-help tips in this book are recommendations that have worked well for many pregnant women. It is important to remember, however, that what works for one person may not work for another. Conversely, because a therapy was not useful to someone else does not necessarily mean that it will not work for you.

If you do have problems during pregnancy it is always advisable to see your doctor first to rule out any serious illness. This is particularly important if you are under medical treatment already. Always discuss any plans you might have for complementary therapy with your doctor so he is aware of what is going on. Nowadays more doctors and midwives are recognising that complementary therapies do have an important role to play in pregnancy. Your doctor might even be able to recommend a therapist. If not try telephoning the professional organisations listed at the end of this book.

Many practitioners are happy to talk over the telephone or at their clinic before starting treatment. Ask about their experience in treating your condition, their success rate, length of the course and fees. Would they consider it appropriate to suggest the names of some patients whom you could contact? Don't forget to check credentials, standards at the clinic and the general attitude of the staff. Look at their bedside manner. Do you feel reassured and trusting? Trust your intuition. Remember always mention to the practitioner that you are or might be pregnant. Be realistic in your expectations and be prepared to take responsibility for your health. This is true for all types of medical care. Many complementary practitioners will give advice and exercises that need to be practised at home daily. Pay for one session at first and try it. If it is unsuitable stop and try something else instead. Try not to use more than two complementary therapies simultaneously. Many therapies complement each other such as acupuncture and osteopathy; others can have unfavourable interactions e.g. homoeopathy and aromatherapy.

If something works for you do tell your doctor or midwife – they might be able to pass this useful information on to their other patients.

We hope the way this book has been organised makes it interesting and will help you to use it as a quick reference.

Have a safe and healthy pregnancy.

Dr Tanvir Jamil
September 2000

Part One

Your Pregnancy

IMPORTANT NOTE
Always tell your doctor or practitioner that you are
or maybe pregnant *before* taking any medicine or
undergoing any treatment.

PREPARING FOR PREGNANCY

It is important to make the most of the months leading up to your baby's conception. The care you give your body now will maximise your chances of having a happy pregnancy, and a strong and healthy baby.

Most couples are advised to start looking after themselves at least three months before they plan to conceive – but six months of looking after yourselves is even better.

There are several reasons for this. First, it takes at least three months to improve the health of the red blood cells, boosting the immune system and strengthening the body against infection, and both the egg and sperm are also at their most vulnerable during the hundred days prior to conception. Making sure your body is in top condition will enhance your chances of a healthy and happy pregnancy – and a strong and healthy baby.

Also, poor nutrition and bad health at the time of conception can hinder your baby's growth, giving rise to potentially serious health problems later in life. In Britain, the national average weight for a newborn is now around 3.6kg (8lb), though anything between 3.5kg (7lb 8oz) and 4.5kg (9lb 9oz) is considered a healthy weight for a newborn baby. But 7 per cent of British babies weigh in at less than 2.5kg (5lb 5oz), the official low birthweight figure.

Low birthweight can be life threatening to a baby – over half of stillbirths and neonatal deaths are among low birthweight babies. Research shows that children tend to perform less well at school if they were small at birth. And, in later life, people who were small at birth are at a greater risk of heart disease, diabetes and stroke.

DIET

What to avoid

While preparing for pregnancy, both you and your partner should:

- avoid taking any drugs without prior consultation with your doctor
- keep alcohol drinking to an absolute minimum
- give up smoking.

Additionally, you should cut down on caffeine. It can reduce your chances of becoming pregnant and some studies have linked high caffeine intake with low birthweight babies. Women preparing for pregnancy should stick to a maximum of four drinks containing caffeine a day.

What to include

Folic acid

From three months before conceiving, increase your intake of folic acid – it's found in fresh, green, leafy vegetables, fortified cereals and bread (check the nutrition labels), meat, oranges and orange juice, and potatoes, and plays a crucial role in the prevention of neural tube defects (such as spina bifida). It's difficult to get the full daily 600mcg recommended for preconception through diet alone. But we tend to get about 200mcg from our diet and a 400mcg tablet is available to make up the deficit. Folic acid supplements are available over the counter to women planning a pregnancy, and free on prescription once you're pregnant.

Calcium

Calcium is obtained from milk and milk products such as cheese and yogurt, tinned fish, such as sardines, where the bones are eaten, green vegetables and beans. Calcium keeps your bones strong and healthy. As bone density seems to diminish during the first three months of pregnancy it is important to 'stock up' prior to pregnancy if possible. The equivalent of one pint of milk a day (680mg calcium) should be enough.

Iron

Iron is found in red meat, pilchards, beans, lentils, nuts, eggs, leafy green vegetables, fortified cereals, bread and dried fruit, especially apricots. Iron is important to prevent you from becoming anaemic prior to and during pregnancy – anaemic women are more likely to have small, premature babies. (NB Liver is a rich source of iron but, because it's so high in vitamin A, it's recommended that you avoid it before and during pregnancy.)

Vitamin C

Vitamin C, which is found in fresh fruit and vegetables, increases the amount of iron you absorb.

Vitamin D

Vitamin D helps you absorb calcium. The body makes vitamin D in response to exposure to sunlight, but dietary sources include oily fish (e.g. salmon, herring and tuna), eggs and milk.

Vitamins B6 and B12

Vitamins B6 – from meat, fish, egg yolk, avocados, seeds and bananas – and B12 – from eggs, dairy produce, meat, fish, marmite and some breakfast cereals – are important in planning and throughout a pregnancy. Vitamin B12 is vital for the production of the genetic material DNA and works with folic acid to prevent neural tube defects. Women whose diet is significantly low in these vitamins are more likely to give birth to low birthweight (i.e. less than 2.5kg (5lb 5oz)) babies.

OTHER CONSIDERATIONS

When planning a pregnancy check your immunity status for rubella and toxoplasmosis. Rubella immunity is checked routinely by your doctor, but, if you may have been exposed to toxoplasmosis (via a cat litter tray, or contact with sheep) this may also be checked for.

It's also advisable to attend for screening if, in the past, either of you has suffered with sexually transmitted diseases or if you've had many sexual partners. Chlamydia and gonorrhoea can lie dormant in the body for many years without symptoms. They can lead to infertility if untreated. And, if you do become pregnant, you risk passing the infection on to your baby.

EXERCISE

Develop a good exercise programme before getting pregnant to help you feel better, increase your stamina, and help make labour and delivery easier. Below are some hints to help you develop a good programme:

- Before starting any new exercise programme, consult your doctor – especially if you've had past medical problems or pregnancy complications.
- Exercise on a regular basis.
- Start gradually and increase what you do as you build up your strength.
- Wear comfortable clothing.
- Avoid contact sports or risky exercise such as water-skiing or riding.
- Allow plenty of time for warming up and cooling down.
- As always, start off slowly and gradually build up the length of your exercise time.

GETTING TO KNOW YOUR FERTILE TIMES

Most women are fertile for two to seven days a month. You can identify these fertile days by getting used to the changes in your cervical mucus or discharge. Fertile mucus is similar to egg white in texture. It is elastic and stretches to form a string, and as well as acting as a sign of fertility it forms a useful slippery passageway for sperm to swim up through the vagina and cervix into the uterus and up to the fallopian tubes – where they wait for an egg to be released.

You may also know you are ovulating when you feel very interested in sex. Many women experience a surge in their libido around the time of ovulation.

You can also learn to recognise a subtle change in your body temperature. Women can identify body temperature changes by taking their temperature first thing in the morning every day. In menstrual cycles in which they ovulate, the temperature rises by a few tenths of a degree during the cycle and stays this high until the next period. This rise occurs a couple of days after ovulation, so a woman can use her temperature chart to identify when ovulation took place – and if the pattern is established over several months she will know when to expect ovulation in the cycle in which she plans to get pregnant. However, temperature charts do not predict actual ovulation.

It is possible that you might experience some kind of pain around the time of ovulation. Ovulation pain (*mittelschmertz*) varies in different women at different times. Many women will go through a fertile lifetime and never have any inkling of the time of their ovulation. Others complain of a bursting type of pain that is mild in degree and duration, while others will suffer a more severe, cramp-like pain every month.

Ovulation kits, available from the chemists, work by detecting luteinizing hormone (LH) in the urine 24–36 hours before ovulation. But the presence of LH is no guarantee that a woman is ovulating, and the kits are also quite expensive.

FERTILITY PROBLEMS

It is the natural expectation of any couple planning a pregnancy that, sooner or later, they will have a baby – and that, with birth control, they will be able to pace their family, choosing when the woman gives birth and how many children she has. But it's not always that easy. It has been calculated that if a fertile couple have intercourse with no contraception on the most fertile day possible, the woman has a one-in-three to one-in-four chance of a baby (the chances of starting a pregnancy are slightly higher, as not all pregnancies come to term). This means that three times out of four, intercourse, even without contraception, will not produce a baby. Doctors expect couples to have been 'trying for a baby' for an average of 6 months before conceiving – and it won't be considered a problem worth further investigation until they have been trying for about 18 months without success.

Even then, there is a strong chance that the couple will conceive naturally without medical intervention. Approximately 70 per cent of couples have conceived after one year of first trying; 80 per cent after 18 months; and 90 per cent after two years.

Your age at trying to conceive can greatly affect your chances of early success. It is estimated that a normally fertile woman under the age of 25 will need, on average, two to three months to conceive. Over the age of 35, she will need six months or longer. One reason it takes longer to become pregnant as a woman gets older is that the quality of her eggs is in gradual deterioration – so she releases fewer eggs that are capable of being fertilised and achieving a pregnancy.

Age is far less of a factor in male fertility. Although the quality of sperm also deteriorates with age, this only becomes significant beyond the age of 60.

It sounds obvious, but the best way to get pregnant is to have sex as often as you can. Although there are only a few days each month when you can conceive, the quality of sperm deteriorates the longer they remain in the body. So there's no benefit in abstaining more than a couple of days in the hope of increasing the number of sperm available when you're ovulating. Eighty-five per cent of women who have regular unprotected sex become pregnant within one year. If you haven't conceived after 12 to 18 months of timed sexual intercourse see your doctor. But go earlier if:

- you have absent or irregular periods, or a history of pelvic inflammatory disease or endometriosis
- you're overweight or underweight
- you're over 35
- your partner's had groin surgery or a testicle injury any time in his life
- either of you has a history of sexually transmitted infection, or drug or alcohol abuse.

About 28 per cent of couples are told they're infertile with no obvious cause because they have not conceived after two years of trying. But 80 per cent of couples who've been trying for three years are likely to conceive in the following 18 months, and even if you've been trying for five years without success, there's still a 30 per cent chance you'll conceive without treatment.

COMPLEMENTARY TREATMENTS FOR INFERTILITY PROBLEMS

Even a long course of complementary treatment is likely to be cheaper than privately-funded assisted conception, and it should enhance your general health and well-being, while avoiding or delaying the need to use drugs or techniques that may have unpleasant side-effects. (All these treatments are discussed further in Part Three.)

Acupuncture

Acupuncture can stimulate the body's natural hormone production, and may help if your failure to conceive is due to a hormonal disorder. There is evidence from at least one trial that acupuncture can help overcome infertility in such cases. This trial studied two groups of 45 women with similar histories of infertility due to hormonal problems. The first group was given acupuncture on the ear (the area linked to fertility), while the second group was treated with hormones. Twenty-two of the acupuncture-treated women became pregnant; 11 after acupuncture, four spontaneously and seven after appropriate medication. Twenty of the hormone group became pregnant, too; five spontaneously and 15 in response to medication. The only side-effects were seen in the women who had hormonal treatment, and the authors of this study considered that acupuncture offered a valuable alternative therapy for female infertility due to hormonal disorders.

Aromatherapy

Aromatherapy might also help in the treatment of male and female infertility. A qualified aromatherapist will take your medical and emotional history, and can also help you with related problems such as endometriosis, heavy or painful periods, and PMS (pre-menstrual syndrome). As well as helping to overcome some infertility problems, aromatherapy offers a pleasant relief from the stress that often accompanies conventional fertility treatments.

Using the oils listed below, some aromatherapists recommend a daily massage over the abdomen, hips, lower back and buttocks, starting on the last day of your period. But remember that the oils can also be used in your bath, in a vapour or on a compress (see page 123).

Rose oil is recommended for regulating the reproductive system. Geranium regulates the menstrual cycle. Bergamot balances hormones. Melissa also regulates the cycle, and has the added bonus of being uplifting – very useful if your fertility problems are getting you down.

Cypress, thyme, nutmeg, coriander, geranium, fennel and Roman chamomile are also beneficial for women trying to conceive.

Regular treatments with thyme, cumin, sage, clary sage and basil are all recommended for male infertility.

Ayurveda

In Ayurveda, asparagus, fenugreek, garlic, onion and liquorice are said to invigorate the reproductive organs. Fenugreek and liquorice should not, however, be taken if you suspect you may be pregnant.

Cranial osteopathy

Although medically unproven and controversial, cranial osteopathy is claimed to be helpful for women with fertility problems. One theory is that, if a trauma or injury has affected the way in which the bones in the head move (you may be completely unaware of this problem), then the pituitary gland controlling your reproductive hormones may be restricted and unable to function properly. In this case, the osteopath's gentle touch may free the movement in the area, and allow the pituitary gland to work normally – although it's impossible to prove how or whether this works. Many cranial osteopaths also work, very gently, on the coccyx, sacrum and other pelvic bones. This can be particularly useful if you have had a previous injury to the area.

Herbal medicine

Herbs have an excellent reputation for enhancing fertility. They appear to do this both by balancing the hormones and by creating a favourable condition in the uterus. Over five hundred plants contain phytoesterols, or plant hormones, which mimic our own hormones. These include natural yam, true unicorn root, false unicorn root, squaw vine, blue and black cohosh. False unicorn root stimulates the ovaries themselves and is considered so potent by herbalists that women wishing to avoid pregnancy are advised not to use it! Natural plant hormones work with human female hormones and are an exciting new discovery in gynaecological medicine. A medical herbalist will prescribe a programme of herbs to prepare you for conception and aid fertility. This programme should be stopped once you become pregnant, and you should not take wild yam, cohosh or false unicorn root if you suspect you may be pregnant. If you want to try some of the gentler herbs known to boost fertility, substituting herbal teas or infusions for coffee and ordinary tea is useful – especially if you are trying to reduce your caffeine intake. Red clover and raspberry leaf contain good levels of minerals, particularly calcium and magnesium, which are thought to aid conception.

(NB See page 134 for herbs contra-indicated in pregnancy. Also as some Chinese herbs contain steroids it would be best to avoid them altogether if you are pregnant or thinking of conceiving. Western herbalism is very safe, but as always do tell the therapist you may be pregnant.)

Homoeopathy

Two studies on the effects of homoeopathy on fertility were published in Germany in 1993. In the first, 21 women with infertility due to hormonal disorders were matched to a similar group of women. One group was treated homoeopathically, while the other was treated with hormonal drugs. Six women in each group became pregnant, and all six from the homoeopathic group went on to have their babies, while four of the hormone group miscarried. In addition to being free of side-effects, the homoeopathic treatment was ten times cheaper than the drug treatment.

There are homoeopathic remedies to treat both male and female infertility. For example, Sepia or Pulsatilla may be prescribed to strengthen a woman's reproductive system; and either sex may be treated with tin, iron or calcium for a chemical imbalance. Sabina 6c may be recommended if you have had previous miscarriages, and Sepia 6c if your problem is linked to irregular periods and an aversion to sex.

Hypnotherapy

Hypnotherapists have proven success in treating unexplained infertility and can also treat spasmodically blocked fallopian tubes by removing the patient's anxieties and enhancing her self-esteem. In 1994 research at the Chelsea and Westminster

Hospital, London, showed that hypnotherapy can reduce stress levels and help some women conceive. It may also help uncover fears about labour, motherhood, hospitals or a baby as a threat to your relationship.

Naturopathy

Naturopaths believe a healthy, balanced diet, regular exercise and a positive attitude are essential for general health and fertility. They suggest you should also avoid caffeine, which is suspected of hindering ovulation, and aim to eat organic fruit and vegetables. Drinking too much alcohol can increase the hormone prolactin, which may disturb your menstrual cycle. Smoking is also seen as harmful, reducing blood flow to your cervix and inhibiting the action of cilia, the tiny hairs in the fallopian tubes that guide the egg towards the uterus. Hot baths should be avoided prior to intercourse as sperm need cool temperatures in order to survive.

Reflexology

Reflexologists claim great success in treating infertility, especially in women. There is little research evidence of this, however, although a small trial in Denmark that recruited women with fertility problems via a newspaper had some interesting results. In all, 108 women started treatment. The average length of time they had been trying to conceive was 6.7 years and their average age was 30.2 years. Forty-seven of the women dropped out during the course of the trial. But, of the remaining 61 who completed a 16-session, 7-month course of treatment, 19 became pregnant within the first six months and 75 per cent of the total experienced an overall improvement in their health.

All the reproductive organ reflexes are situated around the ankle area. These are the ovaries, testes, uterus, prostate, fallopian tubes and vas deferens. See page 165 for illustration.

One of the most important aspects of complementary healthcare is the understanding it gives you of your body. By following the suggestions in this chapter we hope you will feel more confident in yourself as you undergo the very special changes of pregnancy.

2

THE FIRST TRIMESTER

Congratulations on your pregnancy! The first trimester is an exciting time for any mum-to-be. A degree of anxiety is natural, but take any worries in your stride. The majority of women have easy pregnancies, and any minor problems you may encounter can be simply remedied using the tips in this chapter.

From a cluster of cells at conception, it takes just 12 weeks for your baby to develop not just a head, body and limbs, but also ankles, wrists, fingers and toes. By the end of the first trimester she is even producing her own urine. Although she is still only 6.5cm (2in) long and weighs just 18g (¹/₂oz), and your pregnancy may be barely noticeable to others, your body is undergoing enormous changes to accommodate and nurture your growing child, and any symptoms you may have are to do with these changes.

SYMPTOMS AND SOLUTIONS

Anaemia

About 20 per cent of pregnant women suffer with iron-deficient anaemia – and most cases develop around the 20th week, even though you may have been tested for anaemia much earlier in the pregnancy. Literally anaemia means 'lack of blood' and occurs when levels of haemoglobin (the red pigment in the blood that carries oxygen around the body) fall below normal. During pregnancy the volume of blood in your circulation increases by as much as a third. Iron is essential for the production of haemoglobin in the body, and overall an extra 550mg is needed throughout pregnancy – 300mg for your baby, 50mg for the placenta and 200mg to offset the blood lost in childbirth.

The body becomes more efficient at absorbing iron during pregnancy, and this, coupled with the fact that you are not losing blood monthly with your usual periods, means that iron supplements are no longer offered as a matter of routine.

Symptoms of iron-deficiency anaemia include pica (abnormal cravings), pallor, lack of energy, dizziness, headaches, shortness of breath on exercise, and palpitations.

You are at greater risk of anaemia if:

- you've had excessive morning sickness that has interfered with your nutrition
- you have a multiple pregnancy
- you've had several babies close together
- you haven't been eating properly.

With mild iron deficiency there may be no symptoms initially, but as the condition deteriorates, you may develop some of the problems listed above.

The baby is unlikely to be iron deficient, even if you are, as its nutritional needs are met before yours. But there's a slightly increased possibility that the baby will be small or slightly premature if you don't take iron supplements to make up for your deficiency.

Check that your diet contains enough iron-rich foods – meat, poultry, eggs, green, leafy vegetables, sunflower and sesame seeds and wholegrain bread. If you have any reason to suspect you are deficient, ask your doctor or midwife to order a blood test and/or prescribe one of the supplements specially formulated for pregnant women. As a matter of course you will have regular blood tests throughout your pregnancy to check for anaemia.

To help boost your iron levels, take the homoeopathic remedies Ferrum or Ferrum Magneticum 9c. These should help and will certainly do no harm.

YOUR BABY'S DEVELOPMENT IN THE FIRST 12 WEEKS
2 weeks (i.e. 14 days after the first day of your last period): Conception takes place.

Also, raspberry and nettle leaf teas are very rich in minerals, including iron. Avoid raspberry leaf until the third trimester. Nettle is safe to use. Or you could take capsules of burdock or gentian. Naturopaths recommend beetroot and beetroot juice to help build the blood.

Appetite increase

The desire to eat more is normal. Don't fight it – pregnancy is not the time to diet. But do eat sensibly.

From the following groups, try to aim for a variety of foods each day to ensure that you get all the nutrients that you and your baby need.

Bread, other cereals and potatoes

Bread, cereals, rice, pasta, noodles and potatoes are good sources of carbohydrates, protein and B vitamins. They're also low in fat, filling and relatively cheap. Aim for four to six servings per day (one serving is the equivalent of two slices of bread, or a bowl of cereal, or two potatoes, or a portion of rice or pasta).

Fruit and vegetables

Aim to eat four to six servings per day and try to include dark green vegetables such as spinach or broccoli, and orange-coloured vegetables and fruit. Remember:

- always wash fruit and vegetables before you cook and eat them
- don't store fruit and vegetables for too long
- eat some raw vegetables each day
- steaming or microwaving fruit and vegetables is preferable to boiling them, which cooks out a lot of the important vitamin content.

YOUR BABY'S DEVELOPMENT IN THE FIRST 12 WEEKS

3 weeks: The embryo implants in the wall of the uterus. In a week it has grown from one cell to a mass of over a hundred cells and is still growing. The outer cells reach out like roots to link with your blood supply. The inner cells form into two, and then later into three layers, which become different parts of the baby's body. One layer becomes the brain and nervous system, skin, eyes and ears. Another becomes the lungs, gut and stomach, and the third becomes the heart, blood, muscles and bones.

Meat, fish and other sources of protein

Meat, poultry, fish, eggs (cooked thoroughly to avoid salmonella infection), nuts and pulses (baked beans, lentils, chick peas and red kidney beans) are a major source of protein, vitamins and minerals. Aim to eat two to three servings per day. Cook meat and fish right through and avoid pâté.

Dairy products

Milk, yogurt and cheese are high in calcium and also provide protein. Aim for two to three servings per day, but avoid unpasteurised products. One serving is equivalent to one-third of a pint of milk, a small pot of yogurt or $1^{1}/_{2}$oz Cheddar cheese. The low fat varieties offer just as much calcium as their high fat alternatives.

Cheeses best avoided in pregnancy are ripened soft cheeses such as Brie and Camembert, and all blue-veined cheeses (even pasteurised) such as Stilton, Roquefort, Danish blue and dolcelatte.

You can safely eat hard cheeses like Cheddar, Babybel, Gruyère, Edam and Parmesan; and soft cheeses such as Philadelphia, mozzarella and processed cheese spreads.

General advice

- Avoid too many fatty and sugary foods.
- Remove visible fat from meat and take the skin off chicken.
- Grill rather than fry.
- Steam or bake fish for the healthiest results.
- Cut down on fatty butter spreads. Low-fat spreads can taste just as good in a sandwich.
- Keep sweet puddings, biscuits and cakes for occasional treats, rather than having them every day.

YOUR BABY'S DEVELOPMENT IN THE FIRST 12 WEEKS

4 weeks: Eyes and ears start to form, and the baby's head and 'tail' are present.

5 weeks: The arms start to form. The baby already has some of its own blood vessels and a string of these connect the baby to you, forming the umbilical cord.

Bleeding gums

This is caused by increased blood-flow and softening of the gums due to raised levels of the hormone progesterone. Remember to visit your dentist during pregnancy.

Use diluted lemon juice as a mouthwash, or make the following herbal treatment. Combine tincture of marigold (which is antiseptic and healing) with astringent tinctures of agrimony, blood root or bistort. Dilute one part of the tincture in eight parts of warm water and swill in the mouth twice daily, or more if needed.

Breast changes

Especially in your first pregnancy, the growth of your breasts is likely to be one of the first signs of impending pregnancy. Just as some women experience swelling and hardening of their breasts pre-menstrually, the hormones that govern pregnancy have the same effect – though usually more pronounced.

These changes are aimed at preparing you to feed your baby when it arrives. If they are less pronounced in a second or subsequent pregnancy, it doesn't mean that you will be less capable of breastfeeding. Having gone through one pregnancy already, they may need less preparation time (although some women balloon from the first month with every pregnancy) and may gradually grow with your growing baby, or may hold off until after the delivery when milk production begins.

As well as getting bigger – sometimes as much as three cup sizes bigger – your breasts will probably undergo other changes:

- The areola (the pigmented area around the nipple) will darken and spread. This darkening may fade but not disappear entirely after birth.

- The little bumps on the areola may also enlarge. These are sweat glands and return to normal after you've had the baby, or after you've stopped breastfeeding.

YOUR BABY'S DEVELOPMENT IN THE FIRST 12 WEEKS

6 weeks: The spinal canal closes around the spinal cord. If you were to have an ultrasound scan now to confirm the pregnancy, it would be able to pick up the baby's heart movements, and the embryo should be visible.

7 weeks: The head and body are now well established, and the baby is now about 8mm long from head to bottom, though it's too early to see different structures of the embryo on an ultrasound scan.

● Blue veins on your breasts may become more noticeable, but the skin will eventually return to normal.

Especially during the first trimester, your breasts may be agonisingly tender to touch. Fortunately this tends to pass after the 12th week. Soothe sore breasts with warm water compresses (see page 69), or compresses of lavender or damask rose flower water. A comfortably hot bath also relieves painful breasts. Also, for proper support, do make sure you wear well-fitted bras.

Complexion problems

Some women are blessed with a glowing complexion in pregnancy. Others, unfortunately, suffer with acne. Both states are brought about by the increased secretion of oils due to hormonal changes. If you are the type to get pre-menstrual acne, don't get too excited about your face clearing up once you're pregnant – you're as likely to break out in spots now too. The following may help if you suffer complexion problems:

● Stick to your healthy diet, and drink plenty of water to help keep your skin clear.

● Use facial steam baths to open and cleanse the pores, followed by applications of witch-hazel.

● Use the homoeopathic remedy Kali arsenicum (Fowler's solution) 6c, twice a day.

● Drink nettle or dandelion teas. They have a detoxing effect on the body, clearing the toxins that result in spots.

● Echinacea, the immunity-enhancing herb, is safe to use in pregnancy, and should help the cause. Take it as a tincture – 15 drops added to a glass of water.

● Propolis, an antibiotic substance made by bees, can be effective in the form of a cream dabbed on spots.

YOUR BABY'S DEVELOPMENT IN THE FIRST 12 WEEKS
8 weeks: The embryo begins to move and the head can be differentiated from the body on an ultrasound scan. A face is slowly forming. The eyes are more obvious and have some colour in them. There's a mouth with a tongue. There are the beginnings of hands and feet, with ridges where the fingers and toes will be.

(NB: Certain complementary remedies for acne should be avoided in pregnancy. These include wild yam, which is taken orally, and the essential aromatherapy oil of German chamomile.)

Constipation

Constipation is very common in pregnancy. Elimination can be sluggish now that the muscles around the bowel are beginning to relax, and the pressure from your growing womb also inhibits normal bowel activity. Do all you can to avoid being constipated, though, as this can lead to haemorrhoids or piles.

Plenty of fruit and fibre in your diet, washed down with the recommended 4 pints (2 litres) of drinking water every day will help fight constipation. Regular exercise – for example a brisk half-hour walk or a swim – will also help.

Don't worry if you don't get constipated! It's not an obligatory symptom of pregnancy, and, if you don't get constipated, this is most likely to be a sign that you've taken notice and acted upon the previous advice for changing your diet and lifestyle prior to getting pregnant. If your stools are very frequent (more than twice a day) or loose, watery, or containing blood or mucus, you should consult your doctor. Diarrhoea during pregnancy should not be ignored.

If constipation *is* a problem, but you feel you are already getting your full quota of dietary fibre, it may be worth querying the sources of that fibre. Naturopaths see wheat as a less effective source than oatbran, cornbran or psyllium husks. So, try to vary your diet more. If you eat a lot of bread and pasta, try to swap wheat for alternative grains. Rice, rye and corn-based pastas are all available in healthfood shops, and rye bread, rice cakes and oatcakes can be substituted for wheat bread at some mealtimes each week. While increasing fibre, try to cut down on your consumption of meat, dairy products and eggs. If this doesn't work, the following may help:

- Take garlic tablets before bed.
- Soak five or six prunes in cold tea overnight and eat for breakfast with live 'bio' yogurt.

YOUR BABY'S DEVELOPMENT IN THE FIRST 12 WEEKS

9 weeks: Your baby is now about 17mm long from head to bottom. The fingers have separated, but the toes are still stuck together. The arms and legs can be seen on a scan.

- Massage your tummy in a clockwise direction, starting from the left.

- Use the homoeopathic remedies Alumina 6c if you're constipated but have no urge to go to the loo, or Nux Vomica 6c if the reverse is true. If your stools seem to be retreating, take Silica 6c.

- Acupuncture can be helpful. A practitioner will try to restore the natural contractions of the colon, possibly by stimulating acupoints along the Large Intestine and Liver meridians. Acupressure can be practised at home. Lie on your back and gently press the fingertips at a point three finger widths below the navel.

- Many yoga positions are safe in pregnancy and stimulate the gastrointestinal tract to work more smoothly. Tell your yoga teacher you are pregnant, so you can avoid any uncomfortable or inappropriate positions.

- Take *Lactobacillus acidophilus* supplements to increase the bowel flora to break down faeces.

- Use molasses instead of other sweeteners – or take two dessertspoonfuls before bedtime.

Cramp after orgasm

Cramping during and after orgasm is very common and harmless during a low-risk pregnancy. It's caused by congestion of the sexual organs during arousal and orgasm, and venous congestion in the pelvic area. The advice is to take things gently. This might help prevent cramping.

Cravings

Don't expect to start craving coal or disinfectant now you're pregnant. Although it may be a popular idea that this is what happens, there are very few recorded cases of these bizarre cravings (known as pica). And those there are tend to come from research carried out in the 1950s, when women's nutrition was generally not as good as it is now. Pica, if it happens, can be a sign of a nutritional deficiency, particularly of iron, so it should be reported to your practitioner.

YOUR BABY'S DEVELOPMENT IN THE FIRST 12 WEEKS
10 weeks: The heart is fully formed and the embryo is now called a foetus.
It has a human appearance with eyes, eyelids and ears, and looks like a little human on an ultrasound scan.

More common cravings tend to involve ice-cream, chocolate, citrus fruits and juices, and sweets. And some research suggests that women who crave foods in pregnancy are more likely to develop nausea than those who don't. But most women stop suffering with cravings after the first trimester. (See also Food aversions.)

You should stick to your healthy diet. Avoiding too much sugar and fat should help. Certain homoeopathic remedies can also help cravings (see Part Three, Chapter 17).

Dizziness or fainting

Dizziness is common in the first trimester and may be related to the pressure on your blood supply to meet your rapidly expanding circulatory system. You may also feel dizzy if your blood sugar is low because you have gone too long without food. In this case eat something rich in protein at every meal to keep blood sugar stable, and try eating more frequent, smaller meals or snacks between meals. You should also try not to stand up too quickly when you've been sitting or lying, as the sudden shift of blood away from the brain causes dizziness.

Anaemia (see also p.20 and p.11 for dietary advice) can also make you dizzy, as well as tired. If you think you might be anaemic do see your doctor or midwife. Sometimes you may need to take iron tablets to help. These can make you constipated and make your stools look very dark, almost black. To help the constipation try drinking more water (especially on warm days) and increase the amount of fibre in your diet (e.g. bran flakes and brown bread). A particularly good remedy if you do not suffer from heartburn, is a glass of fresh orange juice once or twice daily.

If you think you're going to faint, increase circulation to your brain by lying down, preferably with your feet up. Actual fainting is rare, but if you do faint it won't affect the baby. Recover from fainting by lying down with your feet up, or sitting with your head down between your knees. But report actual fainting promptly to your doctor, or mention any dizziness you've been experiencing at your routine visit.

- If dizziness is a recurrent problem, eat frequent, small, high-protein meals.
- Make sure your clothes aren't too tight around the waist.

YOUR BABY'S DEVELOPMENT IN THE FIRST 12 WEEKS

11 weeks: The spine, skull and some internal organs are now visible on a scan.

● Ginger improves circulation and can relieve dizziness, especially if related to morning sickness. Suck on crystallised or dried (not fresh) ginger, eat a ginger biscuit, or sip ginger beer. If you don't like the taste, take ginger in a capsule form. Ginger is also useful after a fainting incident. Teas of elderflower and rosemary, made with honey and ginger, are also traditional remedies.

● Use the homoeopathic remedy Aconite 6c (four pills every 15 minutes). If you're particularly dizzy when you rise from sitting or lying, take Bryonia 30c (one dose three times a day for five days).

● Massage acupressure points on the arch of each foot, behind the earlobe, and between the nose and upper lip.

● If tension in your neck is affecting the blood supply to your head, thus causing dizziness, an osteopath can gently manipulate the neck and spine. Exercising the neck muscles can also help. Sit in a chair with your hands in your lap. Look straight ahead at first, then gently rotate your head to the left and hold for a count of ten. Repeat to the right. Then try putting your ear on your shoulder – again for a count of ten. Repeat on the opposite side. Finally, put your chin on your chest and hold again for a count of ten. Do this exercise for five minutes, three or four times a day.

● After fainting, put a few drops of peppermint oil on a hanky for gentle inhalation.

Fatigue and sleepiness

Even when you're resting your body is working harder than it ever did before you were pregnant. During this first trimester it's working extra hard to produce the placenta that will be your baby's life support system (and will be complete around the fourth month), so during this time you may need to give in and take more rest than you'd planned. Don't overdo it; fatigue is a sign that your body needs time off. If you are at home without other children to look after, indulge in a regular after-noon nap during the first three months. Even if you can't afford this luxury, you can go to bed an hour earlier at night, and enlist the help of your partner in the morning so you can sleep in. But don't skip exercise because you're tired. A walk will do you good – too much rest and not enough activity will make you even more tired – but don't push yourself too far.

- Avoid sugary foods and caffeinated drinks, as these cause energy highs and lows.

- Evening primrose oil tablets can help counter the effects of fatigue. Take up to six 500mg tablets a day.

- The herbal remedies oats, St John's wort, borage, betony and alfalfa raise the spirits and make you feel generally more energetic. Make an infusion, using 2–4g of any of these herbs to one cup of water, three times daily.

- Proprietary herbal tonics such as Floradix, a combination of iron-rich herbs and vitamins, are recommended for fatigue and safe to use in early pregnancy.

- See also Anaemia, page 20.

Flatulence (wind)

Your windiness will not affect your baby, unless it prevents you from eating regularly and properly, but you can stop it happening, and save yourself a lot of embarrassment, by taking the following measures:

- Fight constipation, as above, page 26.

- Eat six small meals a day instead of three large ones.

- Don't rush your eating.

- Keep calm at mealtimes to avoid swallowing air.

- Avoid culprit foods – onions, beans, cabbage, fried foods, pulses, Jerusalem artichokes, garlic and fizzy drinks.

- Add more fresh ginger to your diet to stimulate your gastric juices and aid digestion.

- Make a dill seed tea, by simmering two teaspoons of seed in a cup of hot water for 15 minutes. The tea will relieve indigestion, heartburn and flatulence. After the birth of your baby, you can carry on drinking it to stimulate the flow of breast milk.

• Fennel and cardamom tea can also help wind. Put half a teaspoon of fennel seeds and one cardamom pod into a cup of boiling water. Simmer for two to three minutes and slip slowly. (NB Drink **no more than** three cups a day.)

Food aversions

Mercifully a lot of women tend to go off the things that are bad for them in pregnancy, such as coffee and alcohol, and this makes keeping off them a whole lot easier. It's more of a problem if you go off healthy foods you know you should be eating. Don't force feed yourself, but do try to compensate with suitable alternatives from the same food group.

If you notice that certain foods smell or taste peculiar now you're pregnant, this could be a sign of zinc deficiency, according to one study, so be aware of that and check that you're including enough zinc-rich foods in your diet (e.g. meat, nuts, oats, potatoes and shellfish).

Frequent urination

Most pregnant women notice that they need to use the loo more than usual – particularly in the first and last trimesters. This is because you're producing a greater volume of body fluids and the kidneys are responding by speeding up the process by which they get rid of the waste products. Also the growing uterus is putting pressure on the bladder while they are still next to each other in the pelvis during the first trimester. You may be relieved from having to go to the loo quite so often once the uterus has risen into the abdominal cavity around the fourth month. In the mean time, try leaning forward when you urinate to make sure you empty your bladder completely. And, to avoid too many trips to the loo at night, try not to drink a lot in the last two hours before bedtime.

If frequent urination is causing real problems, acupuncture, craniosacral work and osteopathy can all help greatly. The homoeopathic remedies Umbellata 6c or Linaria 6c can be taken at a dose of four pills every four hours for a maximum of five days. Pelvic floor exercises (see over) will help tone up the muscles around the urinary exit.

PELVIC FLOOR EXERCISES

The pelvic floor is the sling of muscles that helps hold the pelvis organs in place, and pelvic floor exercises are important throughout your life. If the muscles are allowed to become slack in this area you will enjoy sexual intercourse less and may have more difficulty than before in reaching orgasm. Your partner may also find lovemaking less enjoyable. A particularly weak pelvis floor can lead to incontinence and sagging vaginal walls.

A strong pelvic floor is especially important during pregnancy because the increase in progesterone softens tissues and ligaments and allows the body to stretch more easily. The pelvic floor softens too, and the weight from your growing baby may weaken it. Strengthening the pelvic floor now will help you avoid 'leaking' when you laugh or sneeze after the baby is born, and will also help the vagina to return to normal soon after pregnancy – and enable you to heal faster if you have to have stitches.

You can test the strength of your pelvic floor during intercourse, by squeezing your partner's penis in your vagina; or, when you are urinating, stop the flow and restart it. If you can stop completely in mid-flow, your muscles are in good shape. (But avoid doing this if you suffer regularly with bladder infections.)

The drawbridge exercise – the essential pelvic floor exercise – is best learned when you're lying down.

- Lie down with your knees bent up, hip-width apart, and your feet flat on the floor. Let your arms relax.
- Tighten the vagina as if you're clamping it around a tampon.
- Tighten the urethra as if you're trying to hold back a pee.
- Tighten the anus as if you're trying to hold back a bowel movement.
- Now think of these three tightened areas as one bridge or lift, and imagine you are lifting the drawbridge up inside you: tighten a little, then stop (without relaxing), then tighten a little more and stop again. Hold this squeeze and breathe slowly in and out, then let your drawbridge down in as many stages as you can manage.

Once you've mastered the exercise lying down, you can try it when sitting or standing or walking – and aim to do it whenever you can: every time you make a cup of tea; do the washing up; take the dog for a walk; brush your teeth; or watch a favourite TV show and so on. Getting into a habit will make you do the exercise without even thinking about it. One exercise class for postnatal women got them to do their pelvic floor exercise to the tune of 'Bridge Over Troubled Water'. The argument was that this is still one of the world's most-played records and that women would find themselves doing their exercise while standing in shop queues and sitting in cafes where the song was being played!

Headaches

Pregnancy headaches are commonly caused by hormonal changes, but also fatigue, tension and stress and hunger. Make sure you get plenty of rest and eat regularly.

Give yourself a facial massage to relieve headaches. With your hands in front of your face, palms towards you, use the middle finger pad all along the outer edges of your eye socket zone. (Don't forget to remove your contact lenses first.) With your hands in the same position, bring your middle finger forwards to press up against the bottom edge of the cheekbone, and out to the temple. Keep your eyes shut and afterwards lie down with eye pads soaked in lavender water, and use a hot water compress (see page 69) for the forehead.

For tension headaches, use the homoeopathic remedies Arnica 30c or Ignatia 6c – one dose every 15 minutes of an attack up to a maximum of ten doses. Meditation (see Part Three, Chapter 20) using visualisation and imagery also helps. Neck exercises can also help tension headaches (see page 29 above).

For a migraine, use the reflexology technique of squeezing the tips of your big toes. Also, acupuncture is excellent for migraine and you will probably notice quite a significant improvement after three or four sessions. An acupuncture exercise you can do for yourself for migraine is to press on Liver 2 for two minutes (see Part Three, Chapter 8).

Heartburn

Heartburn is experienced when the ring of muscle that separates the oesophagus from the stomach relaxes, allowing food and harsh digestive juices to travel back up from the stomach to the oesophagus. This is more likely in pregnancy when there is increased pressure on the stomach. These stomach acids irritate the sensitive oesophageal lining, causing a burning sensation about where the heart is – hence the name heartburn, which has nothing to do with your heart.

You will find that it helps to eat small, frequent meals, rather than big, irregular ones. Chew your food thoroughly and avoid eating or drinking too many acid-forming foods like tea, coffee, spicy foods (e.g. curries), sugar, cakes, biscuits, chocolate and artificial sweeteners. Also, avoid alcohol if you have not already done so, and give up smoking completely as both can increase the amounts of acid in your stomach.

Eating more fruit and vegetables can help to neutralise stomach acid. Juicing is an excellent way of increasing your intake. Try apples, carrots and broccoli. Avoid drinking with your meal, but have a drink half-an-hour afterwards – a herbal tea such as peppermint (maximum three cups daily), lemon balm or lemon verbena after meals is particularly helpful.

Papaya and pineapple are both well-known aids to digestion. Try to eat them at some point in the day, or chew two or four papaya enzyme or pineapple bromelain tablets with a meal.

Indigestion

Early in pregnancy your body produces large amounts of progesterone and oestrogen. These relax the muscles everywhere, including the gastrointestinal tract, and this can cause food to move more slowly through your system – leading to bloating and indigestion. Although uncomfortable for you, the slow-down of the digestive process allows better absorption of nutrients into your bloodstream and subsequently the placenta, which feeds your baby, so you can console yourself that, while you may hate the results, they're in a good cause.

Better posture, achieved with the Alexander Technique, can help a lot. Also, the homoeopathic remedies Capsicum 6c, Carbo Vegetabilis 6c or Asafoetida 6c can be taken three or four times a day to ease indigestion.

10 WAYS TO AVOID HEARTBURN AND INDIGESTION

1. Avoid gaining too much weight – it will put more pressure on your stomach.
2. Wear loose clothing, so your stomach isn't squeezed.
3. Eat six small meals rather than three large ones.
4. Eat slowly, taking small mouthfuls and chewing them thoroughly.
5. Avoid fried and fatty foods, processed meat (e.g. sausages and bacon), chocolate, coffee, alcohol and fizzy drinks.
6. Don't smoke.
7. Relax as much as you can.
8. Sleep with your head supported – use an extra pillow or put a firm block under your pillow, or elevate the head of your bed by putting a brick under the top two legs.
9. Bend at the knees instead of the waist.
10. The commonly available antacids available from your pharmacist, Gaviscon and Mixture of Magnesium Trisilicate, are safe in pregnancy.

Libido changes

If you've never had an enormous appetite for sex you may be surprised at how it has increased since becoming pregnant. Feeling sexier is one of the nicest symptoms many women experience, but it may not happen until the second trimester (see Chapter 3), especially if you suffer with nausea, excess fatigue, and painful breasts in the first 12 weeks.

Milk intolerance

Many women go off milk in pregnancy. Don't worry if it happens to you. Although you need calcium for your baby, it does not have to come from milk – try cheese and yogurt, or tinned fish like sardines, where you eat the bones, green vegetables and beans. If you can't tolerate any of these, talk to your doctor about taking a supplement.

Nausea

Over 80 per cent of pregnant women suffer from some level of morning sickness. It's thought to be caused by chemical by-products of increased hormonal activity building up and creating general toxicity in the body. But nobody knows why some women are affected while others are not.

In its most severe form – Hyperemesis gravidarum – women vomit so much that they cannot keep even a sip of water down, and have to be fed fluids intravenously. If you are vomiting a lot, it's essential you consult your doctor for advice, as the condition can become life-threatening to you and your baby.

Treatments include: getting as much rest as possible (nausea may be your body's way of telling you to take it easy); taking your time to get out of bed in the morning; indulging your cravings; getting plenty of exercise and fresh air; and separating drinks from meals. Avoid cooking as far as possible. Steer clear of fried foods and caffeine. And don't brush your teeth straight after a meal as this can make you gag. Some other remedies are listed below:

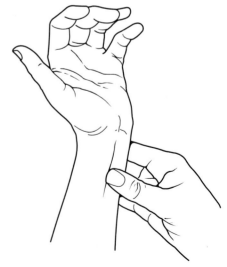

- The acupressure points for nausea are at the base of the wrist, Pericardium 6, (see Part Three, Chapter 8). Press on these for several seconds to relieve nausea. A study showed a 60 per cent improvement in morning sickness in women who used acupressure like this. You can also buy acupressure bands to do this job for you, and are just as effective for travel sickness. Acupuncture can help with severe vomiting. A session twice a week for three or four weeks may ease your vomiting considerably.

- Dry crackers can also help ease the feeling of nausea first thing in the morning.

Acupressure points on the wrist

● Ginger supplements have been proven to ease nausea by helping food pass more rapidly through the digestive system, as well as reducing the stimulation to the part of the brain that prompts a burst of nausea or vomiting. Keep a ginger biscuit by your bed to nibble first thing in the morning.

● Try sipping water of fizzy drinks throughout the day. During a bout of nausea, sip a cup of peppermint tea.

● The homoeopathic remedies Ipecac 6c, Sepia 6c, Pulsatilla 6c, Nux Vomica 6c can also help. Take one tablet three to four times daily until you feel an improvement.

● The Bach flower remedy Crab Apple is also very useful for sickness at any time of day.

● Adding a few drops of lavender oil to your bath water has an anti-emetic effect. Other aromatherapy oils to try are chamomile, rose and ginger.

● Try Ayurvedic coconut water: add one teaspoon of fresh lemon juice to the fresh juice of a coconut and sip every 15 minutes to settle your stomach.

● Soak ten raw (unroasted) almonds overnight, and the next morning peel off the skins and eat them. They provide high quality protein and calcium, both of which you need – and also settle the stomach.

● Drink as much as you can to compensate for vomiting, which can lead to dehydration. A useful drink to keep by your side is a pint of water mixed with two teaspoons of sugar, the juice of half a lime, and a pinch of salt. Try to drink a cup of this every two hours to prevent dehydration and help the sickness subside.

● Go for a walk. Ayurvedic practitioners recommend walking, as getting a bit of fresh air will reduce 'pitta' and relieve stress (see Part Three, Chapter 13). The idea behind this is that a 'pitta' woman may develop unresolved anger. The stress of this builds up in the solar plexus, and manifests itself as morning sickness.

Saliva

You may find you produce excessive saliva during the first trimester. This is known as ptyalism, and can be so bad that it's impossible to swallow the amount of saliva produced without being sick. It is more common in women experiencing morning sickness than those who aren't, but usually disappears after the first few months.

If it's a problem, and is making you sick, use the remedies suggested for nausea above.

Sleeping difficulties

It's one of the ironies of early pregnancy that, despite increased fatigue during the day, you find you cannot sleep well at night. The following tips may help:

- Develop a bedtime routine, with a slow pace after dinner and a relaxing bath before bed. Try to go to bed at the same time every night.

- Don't take work to bed with you; it will make your mind race and prevent you sleeping. Instead, read something light or listen to soothing music.

- Naturopaths associate iron deficiency with poor sleep. An iron-rich diet, with plenty of pulses, dark green leafy vegetables and nuts, can help.

- Too much caffeine is a classic culprit for a restless night, so try to avoid too much coffee, tea, chocolate or cola in the evening.

- Going to bed feeling hungry, or too full, will keep you awake. Try to eat early in the evening and, if you're hungry just before bedtime, eat something sleep-inducing like a banana.

- A sweetened milk drink at bedtime will help you sleep because the sugars enable the brain cells to absorb more tryptophan (provided by the milk protein) from the bloodstream. This is then converted into serotonin, which is calming.

- Starch foods – pasta, rice and potatoes – balance blood sugar levels and also encourage the release of serotonin.

- If you really can't sleep, don't lie there thinking about it. Get up and do something to take your mind off it, such as reading, watching TV or knitting. When you feel sleepy go back to bed and try again.

- Acupuncture can help enormously.

- The aromatherapy oil neroli can also aid sleep. Put a few drops on your pillow.

- If your problem is that you wake in the night and can't get back to sleep, try the homoeopathic remedy Cocculus 6c or Kali Phosphoricum 6c. Take two or three doses hourly before bedtime.

● Gentle sedative herbs such as lime flower, passion-flower, skullcap, lemon balm, orange blossom, rose petal or chamomile are useful. Take them in tea during the day, as well as the evening, making an infusion of 2–4g of each herb (any combination) in one cup of water, and drink three cups daily and one or two at bedtime. Use honey to sweeten the tea as this also aids sleep. A stronger sedative, valerian, should be avoided in the first trimester.

Venous changes

Blue lines on your breasts and abdomen are normal – they are a sign that your body is doing what it should and expanding its network of veins to carry the increased blood supply required in pregnancy. They may be especially noticeable if you're very slim or pale skinned.

Thread veins – purplish red lines, usually on the thighs – can result from the hormone changes in pregnancy and often fade after delivery. If the thread veins have not faded six months after delivery they can be removed by injecting the vein or by destroying it with a weak laser beam. These procedures need to be carried out by a surgeon at hospital but are usually only available privately. This is because thread veins by themselves are considered to be only a cosmetic problem.

Varicose veins affect about 15 per cent of adults – and mostly women. The disorder tends to run in families and usually the veins appear on the backs of your calves or the insides of your legs when they're blue and visibly enlarged. Where the vein is prominent you may get a severe ache, especially if you've been standing a long time, your feet and ankles may swell, and your skin is likely to be itchy. These symptoms are often extra bad in pregnancy, and sitting with your legs up is the best way to ease any discomfort.

Varicose veins are caused by pooling of blood in the superficial veins when the valves that normally prevent blood from draining back down the leg are defective – and the hormonal changes in pregnancy and pressure from your enlarged uterus can contribute to this happening.

You should be able to treat the condition by wearing support stockings, walking regularly, standing still as little as possible and sitting with your feet up when you're resting. Getting plenty of vitamin C is supposed to keep veins healthy and elastic.

Swollen 'varicose' veins can occur around the vulva in pregnancy. To avoid them, try not to sit with your legs crossed or stand for long periods, and try to avoid putting on too much weight. Sleeping with your legs on a pillow can help.

Massaging veins gently with diluted cypress oil will help to shrink them. You could also add a few drops of lemon and cypress oils to your bath water. If you don't have cypress oil, but want a gentle massage, use a moisturising cream such as E45. Also, horse chestnut extract is an excellent remedy for varicose veins on the legs and has been used on the continent for years. Do not rub it in as it may cause inflammation, but apply very gently to strengthen the fibrous tissue supporting the veins. Vitamin E and garlic will both help, too. Take 300–600IU vitamin E, and one to six garlic perles daily.

If your legs ache and feel bruised and strained, take the homoeopathic remedy Arnica 6c or Bellis Perennis 6c, three times daily.

Waistline expansion

If you started out very slim, your waistline may begin to expand very early in pregnancy as you have little excess flesh for your growing uterus to hide behind. But it could be a sign that you're gaining too much weight too soon. If you've put on 3lb (1.4kg) by the second month, take a look at your diet and cut out any empty calories (i.e. cakes, sweets etc.).

Weight gain

Some weight gain is normal, but not obligatory, in the first three months. Even if morning sickness has prevented you gaining any weight, your baby will be OK, as its need for calories and certain nutrients now is not as great as it will be later. But not gaining weight from the end of the third month onwards can have an effect. So try to eat well from now on, aiming to gain 1lb (approximately $\frac{1}{2}$kg) a week through to your eighth month.

If you've gained too much weight in your third month, there's little you can do about it now. Dieting is not an option in pregnancy. But eat sensibly, cutting out the fatty puds and junk food, from now on.

With all the changes that have been taking place in these first 12 weeks it may seem amazing that your pregnancy is only now becoming visible to the outside world. As you prepare to enter your middle trimester, look forward to regaining your energy and watching your baby grow.

3

THE SECOND TRIMESTER

Make the most of your body now – enjoy good posture and try some of the herbal and aromatherapy suggestions in this chapter. Many will enhance your general feeling of well-being.

The second trimester is well known for being the 'energetic phase' of pregnancy – but don't enter it expecting to feel more energetic than you did before the pregnancy! Although your body is less tired now that it has got through the strenuous first weeks of manufacturing the baby, and morning sickness may also be subsiding, a lot of your energy is still going towards nurturing your baby, who is finally making its presence felt in fluttery movements – although in fact it has been moving around, undetected to you, since the seventh week.

Ironically, it is often during this momentous phase of the pregnancy, that some mums-to-be start to have their first misgivings about the imminent disruption to their lives. Studies show that not only is a little ambivalence, or even fear, normal, it's also quite healthy – as long as these feelings are confronted. This is a good time to talk any worries through with your partner, and work out how you will deal with your new life as a family instead of as a couple.

SYMPTOMS AND SOLUTIONS

Abdominal pain

Most pregnant women experience some degree of abdominal pain with the stretching of the muscles and ligaments supporting the uterus. It may be a sharp or crampy pain, and is often most noticeable when you are standing up after sitting or lying, or when you cough. Mention any pain to your doctor or midwife at your next appointment, but there's no need to seek urgent medical help, unless the pain is persistent or accompanied by other symptoms, such as fever, bleeding, vaginal discharge or faintness.

Chamomile, lemon balm and lime blossom tea can help. You can make your own using 2–4g of each herb per cup. Cramp bark is also very useful. You can buy this in capsule or tablet form, or as a tincture or tea. If you're making your own tea, use one teaspoon of the chopped herb per cup of boiling water. Cover and leave to infuse for five to ten minutes, strain and add honey if desired. Do not add milk or sugar.

For groin pain, practise yoga squats to loosen the hips and pelvic floor. Squat down, keeping your back lengthened. If you can, keep your heels on the floor and balance your weight evenly between the balls of your feet and the heels, not allowing your feet to roll inward or outward. Press your arms against your thighs to increase the stretch on the groin and inner thighs. Start by squatting against a wall, or holding hands with your partner (facing each other).

You may want to squat in labour, and if you've become used to doing this in pregnancy, it won't be too difficult. It also strengthens your thighs and feet, and stretches your Achilles' tendons, calves and inner thigh muscles. Afterwards, always get up slowly, preferably holding on to a chair or table, or you may feel dizzy.

Backache

Backache in pregnancy is one of the side-effects of your joints loosening up so you will be able to deliver your baby. Correcting your posture will help prevent and minimise unnecessary pain, and try the following remedies.

- Swimming is excellent exercise for your back – but avoid breast stroke unless you keep your head in the water, as holding your neck up puts more strain on your back.

- The yoga exercise 'The Cat' is especially good for the lower back (see overleaf).

YOUR DEVELOPING BABY

14 weeks: The foetus is fully developed and about 7.5cm (3in) long from head to bottom. It's still impossible to make out the baby's sex on an ultrasound scan, even though the sex organs are well developed.

THE CAT

Begin on your hands and knees.
Keep your hands just in front of
your shoulders, your legs
hip-width apart. Inhale gently.

As you inhale tilt your pelvis up and let the
spine curve down as you lift your head.

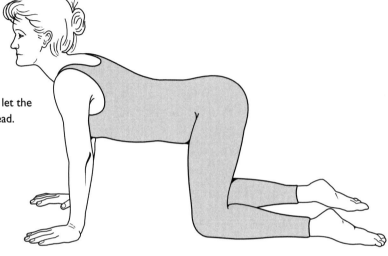

As you exhale, tilt your pelvis down
and draw the spine up pulling your chest and
stomach in, dropping your head.

Repeat several times flowing smoothly
between the two positions.

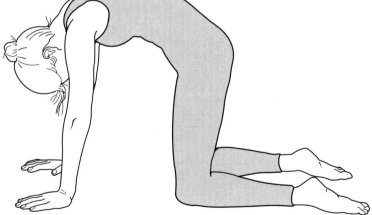

YOUR DEVELOPING BABY

15th and 20th weeks: Between these weeks the baby's body is growing quite rapidly so that the head and body are in better proportion, and the baby doesn't look so top heavy. The face begins to look more human and the baby's hair, eyebrows and eyelashes are all beginning to grow. Toe- and fingernails are growing and the baby has a firm hand grip.

HEALTHY POSTURE

The best way to get out of bed

Stretch the length of your body, bend your knees and roll on to the side you get up from. Stay there for a few moments, then slowly come up to a sitting position with your legs over the side of the bed. Place your feet on the floor and gently push with your hands to lift yourself up.

The best way to stand at a work surface

Stand on both feet, hip-width apart, with your legs straight and your weight evenly distributed. Avoid stooping by bringing the work surface to the right height for you (use a thick chopping board to raise it towards you, or use the table if you're very short). This will help you keep your spine erect and your upper chest free to breathe.

The best way to sit at a desk

Keep your feet or table at the correct height for you to work without slumping forward. Your feet should be on the floor, a little apart, and your knees should be lower than your hips. A wedge cushion on your chair will help (but isn't essential) to push your spine into the correct position, so that you do not sink into your pelvis. If you don't want to buy a wedge, imagine your pelvis as a bowl of water and keep it in a position whereby the water will remain level. Doing this will push your spine up straight, keeping your chest open so you can breathe and work in comfort.

The best way to stand comfortably

Keep your feet slightly apart and your legs straight, with your hands by your side or behind you (which helps you to roll your shoulders back and open your upper chest so you can breathe easily).

The best way to walk

With your spine and head erect, look straight ahead. Wear flat, comfortable shoes, carry your bag across your body, or distribute the weight between bags so both hands are balanced. Roll your shoulders back and down towards your waist, without bending your spine backwards.

The best way to relax in front of the TV

Using the back of the sofa or a block of cushions, support your spine, neck and head so they remain in one line and aren't twisted or slumping. Keep your feet up in front of you, to make you more comfortable, and make sure your shoulders aren't rounded so you can breathe deeply to help you relax.

- Back massage with herbal oils can give local relief. St John's wort oil relieves pain and irritation of the nerve endings.

- The homoeopathic remedies Aesculus 6c and Kali Carbonicum 6c taken one tablet three times a day are beneficial.

- Add a few drops of Arnica mother tincture to bath water to soothe aches and pains.

- Acupuncture over the point Bladder 23 for one to two minutes three or four times a day can also bring relief (see page 113).

- Acupuncture helps relieve severe back pain in pregnancy.

- The Alexander Technique (Part Three, Chapter 9) and Pilates (Part Three, Chapter 23) are both extremely useful in helping relieve back pain and restoring correct posture in pregnancy.

- If back pain is persistent, it may be worth consulting an osteopath or reflexologist.

Blood pressure variations

A 'normal' blood pressure reading is about 120/80. The first figure, the systolic, measures the pressure inside the arteries the instant the heart beats. The second figure, the diastolic, measures the pressure in the arteries when the heart is resting. If your systolic measurement is 140 or higher and the diastolic is 90 or higher you have high blood pressure (hypertension).

It's normal for your blood pressure to change slightly in pregnancy – it often goes down in the second trimester and rises in the third.

Low blood pressure (hypotension) may be supine hypotension, meaning the enlarging uterus is putting pressure on the large blood vessels, e.g. the aorta and the vena cava – and may be most noticeable when you're lying on your back. Or it may be postural hypotension, meaning your blood pressure drops as you rise from sitting. The main symptom is dizziness, but hypotension can be avoided by not sleeping or lying on your back, and rising slowly when you get up.

High blood pressure (hypertension) is worrying as it can be a sign of pre-eclampsia in the second half of pregnancy. A study at St Thomas's Hospital has found that a supervised course of vitamin C and E supplements in the second half of pregnancy is likely to prevent pre-eclampsia. The theory is that the condition is more likely to present if you have run your essential vitamins down during the course of the pregnancy. However, many women develop high blood pressure in pregnancy without pre-eclampsia. Drinking lots of water, avoiding salt, and taking plenty of bed rest can help bring high blood pressure down, and it's important to follow your

---

YOUR DEVELOPING BABY

22 weeks: At about this time the baby becomes covered in very fine hair, known as 'lanugo', which is thought to keep the baby at the right temperature. Usually this hair disappears before birth, but sometimes a little is left – especially on the ears and back – and disappears when the baby is a few weeks old. The baby is now around 25cm (10in) long.

doctor or midwife's advice about this. If they're concerned, you may be admitted to hospital for enforced bed rest where your blood pressure can be monitored every few hours, and you may also be prescribed drugs to lower your blood pressure.

Garlic powder tablets have been proven to lower raised blood pressure and there's anecdotal evidence that fresh garlic works best at lowering blood pressure when combined with watercress – so add both to your salad.

- Flotation therapy can significantly lower raised blood pressure, and also helps you to relax.

- Hyperventilation (overbreathing) can push your blood pressure up – so learn deep breathing exercises and try to breathe from your abdomen. Once your baby is born, you will see breathing at its natural best, as you watch your infant's tummy pump up and down as she breathes!

- Colour therapy uses blue or indigo to lower blood pressure.

- The homoeopathic remedy Kali Chlor. is good for hypertension – although it would be wise to consult a practitioner before self-prescribing.

- Acupuncture has been shown to reduce blood pressure. In women who are being continuously monitored, the digital display shows a fall in blood pressure during acupuncture treatment.

- Aromatherapists use oils of lavender, sandalwood and rose, all of which have sedative qualities.

- Calcium, magnesium and vitamin B6 can all help. A 50mg supplement of vitamin B6 and six Dolomite tablets for calcium and magnesium are recommended.

- The herbal diuretic dandelion is also effective – try a dandelion infusion twice a day, or eat raw or cooked dandelion leaves.

GARLIC AND HIGH BLOOD PRESSURE: THE EVIDENCE SO FAR

The *Journal of Hypertension* reported in 1997 that garlic powder tablets could reduce systolic blood pressure by 10 per cent and diastolic blood pressure by 6 per cent. The journal went on to say that the potential blood pressure lowering effect was of such significance that stroke may be reduced by 30–40 per cent and coronary heart disease by 20–25 per cent. The authors, Professor Christopher Silagy and Dr Andrew Neil, working at the Radcliffe Hospital in Oxford looked at all the published data on garlic and blood pressure, and conducted a review using strict guidelines only to include studies that were properly designed and conducted. Overall, 415 subjects had been studied and they had all been treated with the same powdered garlic tablets (Kwai). The results showed that both systolic and diastolic blood pressure were significantly reduced.

- Qigong (see Part Three, Chapter 28) and T'ai Chi Ch'uan (see Part Three, Chapter 28) are both easy-to-learn active methods of stress control, which can promote a feeling of inner calm and help to keep blood pressure under control.

- Yoga and the Alexander Technique, practised regularly, may also help to lower high blood pressure.

(NB None of the above should be used in place of a doctor's prescription if your doctor advises hypertensive drugs.)

Breathlessness

Severe breathlessness, with rapid breathing and chest pain and/or a rapid pulse and bluish lips or fingers is of concern, and you should call your doctor or go to casualty.

Mild breathlessness is a common experience in the second trimester, caused by hormonal influences swelling the capillaries in the respiratory tract, and relaxing the muscles of the lungs and bronchial tubes. Later in pregnancy, when your uterus is bigger and pushing up against the diaphragm the lungs become more restricted and can't expand fully – but this type of breathlessness is also quite normal.

Frankincense essential oil in your bath can help your breathing. Meditation (Part Three, Chapter 20) and visualisation can also help calm the nerves, ease stress and help with mild breathlessness. Marja Putkisto, a dance and movement specialist, has developed the following deep breathing exercises, which will help you breathe more efficiently. You will find that by practising them, you will achieve a greater sense of relaxation and general well-being. Try to emphasise your exhalation, and always pause between your inhalation and exhalation.

Balloon breathing – focusing on your diaphragm

1. Lying on your back, with your knees bent and feet and knees hip-width apart, lift your pelvis 5–12.5cm (2–5in) off the floor by tilting your tailbone towards your navel.

YOUR DEVELOPING BABY

Weeks 23 to 28: The baby is moving more vigorously and will jump at an unexpected loud noise. It is swallowing small amounts of amniotic fluid, and passing tiny amounts of urine. The baby may also begin to develop a waking and sleeping pattern.

2. Try to drop the weight of your chest towards the base of your ribs, between your shoulder blades.

3. As you breathe in through your nose, visualise your diaphragm moving towards your pelvis, and allow the pressure of your inbreath to bring your abdomen out like a balloon.

4. Breathe out by opening your mouth, releasing your diaphragm and allowing the air to puff out of your lungs.

Rising sun breathing – focusing on your upper lungs

1. Lying on your back, slightly tilt your chin down to lengthen the back of your neck.

2. Place one hand on your chest, fingers up, and the other on the back of your neck, fingers reaching towards the middle of the shoulderblade area.

3. Breathe in through your nose, allowing your breastbone to lift and expand as your lungs fill. Pause. Then breathe out slowly. Pause, then inhale again.

Half moon breathing – focusing on your lower lungs

1. Choose any comfortable position, sitting or lying down. Place your hands on your lower ribcage and keep your upper body and shoulders relaxed.

2. Breathe in, allowing your ribs to expand sideways against your hands. Pause, then slowly breathe out through your mouth keeping your lips firm.

3. As you breathe out, your diaphragm will lift. As you sense it rise, try to squeeze more air out of your lungs.

4. Pause. Then repeat the exercise, this time concentrating on the contraction of your muscles around your ribcage with each outbreath.

For help in a panic attack, where you are gasping with hyperventilation, simply put a small paper bag around your nose and mouth, and breathe in the same air for a couple of minutes, while trying to relax.

YOUR DEVELOPING BABY

24 weeks: The baby is 'viable' – i.e. it now has a chance of survival if it is born prematurely. Before 24 weeks, the lungs and other vital organs are rarely strong enough to cope with life outside the womb. The baby is covered in a white, greasy substance called vernix that protects its skin while it floats in the amniotic fluid. Some of this vernix may still be present at birth.

Chloasma

Often known as 'the mask of pregnancy', chloasma is a dark colouration of the skin on your face and is due to hormonal factors.

The common daisy has a reputation for clearing this type of skin discolouration. Make it as an infusion (2–4g per cup of water) and dab it on to your skin.

Foods rich in PABA (para amino-benzoic acid) are also thought to help. These include wheatgerm, whole grains, mushrooms, fresh fruit and vegetables. Liver is also rich in PABA, but is not recommended during pregnancy because of its high vitamin A content.

Diabetes

Diabetes is caused by a lack of the hormone insulin, which maintains normal amounts of sugar in your blood. As a result your sugar level rises, and this can cause problems for you, and especially your baby.

The hormonal changes you experience in pregnancy increase your blood sugar levels, and most pregnant women produce extra insulin to cope with these increases. However, in some, especially those who are overweight, this is not effective and the blood sugars will start to rise in advancing pregnancy.

In some hospitals routine blood tests may be taken at 28 and 36 weeks of your pregnancy. These include a blood sugar test. In other units, between the 24th and 28th week of your pregnancy a blood test will be taken one hour after a sweet drink has been consumed.

Getting a diagnosis is important as elevated blood sugar levels in pregnancy are associated with an increased risk of complications, especially to your baby, but treatment reduces these risks.

Maintaining normal blood sugar levels in pregnancy will reduce the risk of these complications. And most pregnant women who have diabetes can do this by improving their eating habits. If this is not sufficient, you will need a course of insulin injections for the remainder of the pregnancy.

General advice is to avoid sugar and sweet foods, and eat more high-fibre carbohydrates, e.g. pasta, rice and pulses. Also, limit the amount of fat you eat, and eat at regular times.

Yoga can help reduce stress and enhance pancreatic function. Ayurvedic practitioners may recommend panchakarma, a purification process thought to cleanse the digestive tract and increase vitality. 'Bitter' foods such as green bananas are also thought helpful.

Forgetfulness

Forgetting appointments, feeling as if you're losing brain cells, and experiencing problems concentrating on tasks are normal in pregnancy, and are caused by hormonal changes. Recognising that it's normal should help you through what is, after all, a temporary phase. But to minimise the disruption to your life and stop you stressing yourself out worrying about whether you've remembered to do everything you're supposed to, get into the habit of writing yourself 'To Do' lists, and ticking off the tasks as you go.

The homoeopathic remedy Nux Moschata 6c three times daily may help.

Haemorrhoids (see Rectal bleeding)

Itching

An itchy abdomen is normal in pregnancy – and you may have to apply calamine lotion to stop yourself scratching too much. Itchy limbs are **not** normal, however – and may be the first sign of obstetric cholestasis, a liver condition that can seriously jeopardise your baby's health. Do not ignore itching of the limbs and ask your doctor for a liver function test if it becomes a problem.

Itchy genitals are not uncommon in pregnancy, as you are extra sweaty. Keep yourself very clean, and use a pad soaked in flower water (e.g. rose water) to cool the area.

Leg cramps

The second and third trimesters are often disrupted by leg cramps that can propel you out of bed in the middle of the night. These may be due to excess phosphorus and too little calcium in the blood (maybe due to the fact that as the baby grows it takes more calcium from you), in which case reducing your phosphorus intake (less meat and milk) and increasing your calcium from other food sources (e.g. kelp, white bait, sardines, dried figs, watercress and cooked egg yolks) may help. Calcium supplements should be avoided as they're not well absorbed. Taking half a teaspoon of cider vinegar in water before meals will increase the hydrochloric acid in your stomach and help with the absorption of calcium from your food.

Pressure of the growing uterus on the nerves can be another cause of leg cramps and alternating periods of exercise with periods of rest during the day may help relieve the pain at night.

If you do suffer an attack of cramp, try to straighten your leg and slowly flex your toes and ankle towards your nose. If you can't get rid of the pain, see your doctor. A continuous pain in the calf may be a sign of a blood clot, which needs medical treatment.

- Massaging vigorously helps, or try pressing your hands flat against a wall, keeping your feet flat on the floor about 1m (3ft) away, and putting a good pressure on your hands until the cramp passes.

- The herbal treatment cramp bark specifically helps with this problem. Take one cup two or three times daily with one cup before bed (one teaspoon of the chopped herb per cup of water). A herbal practitioner may also recommend rubbing your legs with a lotion containing cramp bark.

- A bedtime bath can help prevent nightcramps. Add lavender oil to the water, or massage your legs after the bath, using oil to which a few drops of marjoram have been added.

- The homeopathic remedy Magnesium Phosphoricum is also helpful. Crush three tablets in warm water and sip.

Low-lying placenta

The risk of a low-lying placenta is that you will have 'placenta praevia' which puts you in danger of a haemorrhage and makes vaginal delivery almost always impossible, because the placenta is so low it's covering the os, or opening of the uterus. Having said that, 20 to 30 per cent of placentas are moderately low in the second trimester – and the majority move into the upper segment of the womb, where they should be, as the mum-to-be approaches her delivery date. You will be scanned regularly while the placenta is low, especially if you've had any slight bleeding, and may be advised to take plenty of rest and avoid doing anything remotely strenuous until after you have the all-clear.

Painful hands

Another side-effect of swelling in pregnancy is carpal tunnel syndrome. The carpal tunnel in the wrist becomes swollen and this puts pressure on the nerve running through it to your fingers. The pain can radiate up your arm and down through your fingers, and is often more severe at night. If you wake with pain in your hands at night, dangle them over the side of the bed and shake them vigorously. If they're still painful, investigate wearing a wrist splint, which can bring a lot of relief.

An osteopath can manipulate the area to increase mobility and disperse excess fluids in the local soft tissue. An acupuncturist may insert needles into local points around the wrist to help relax tension in the soft tissues.

Perineal pressure

This can increase as your baby grows and presses on the perineum. Lying on your side can help relieve the pressure, and massaging the area with sweet almond oil, then applying a lavender flower water pad, is soothing.

Rectal bleeding and piles

Rectal bleeding in pregnancy is most likely to be a sign of haemorrhoids (piles), which are varicose veins of the rectum, and can cause itchiness and pain. Another cause may be fissures – cracks in the anus caused by constipation, but these are usually extremely painful. Either way, see your doctor to confirm the diagnosis and get advice on treatment. In addition to anything the doctor offers, you can:

- avoid getting constipated
- avoid long hours of standing or sitting
- sleep on your side to relieve pressure on your bottom
- apply witch-hazel compresses or ice packs to ease the pain
- keep your perineal area very clean
- only use topical medications or suppositories prescribed by your doctor for use in pregnancy.

Cypress oil can shrink piles – put a few drops in your bidet or a bowl of warm water and sit in it for as long as you are comfortable. Use the herbal remedy pilewort, which you can buy as an ointment cream from healthfood shops, or tincture of witch-hazel, available through herbal suppliers. The homoeopathic remedies Horse Chestnut 6c, Poison Nut 6c, Peony 6c and Sulphur 6c are also recommended for piles.

Swollen feet and ankles

Normal fluid retention and weight gain can make your feet fuller than they were before pregnancy. This is exacerbated by the hormone relaxin loosening the foot joints (along with other joints), as it starts to loosen the pelvis in preparation for delivery. Any swelling will go down after you've had your baby, but some women find that their joints never fully tighten up, leaving them with feet up to a full shoe size bigger for life. Try some of the following remedies to help your swollen feet and ankles.

- wear comfortable, low-heeled shoes in leather or canvas (to allow your feet to breathe) to make yourself more comfortable
- take regular, gentle exercise to keep the fluids and blood pumping along your circulation
- massage with geranium oil can help fluid retention in pregnancy
- fennel has some diuretic properties and fennel tea can be sipped throughout the day (NB drink **no more than** three cups a day)
- gently massaging your feet, ankles and lower legs can also eliminate some of the fluid.

Vaginal discharge

The normal increase in vaginal discharge or secretion in pregnancy is called leucorrhoea, and is white or creamy coloured and fairly thick. It's caused by the increased blood flow to the skin and muscles around the vagina, which also causes the blue colouration to your vagina ('Chadwick's sign') in early pregnancy. If the discharge is very heavy, wear sanitary towels for protection and avoid nylon underwear. But do **not** douche your vagina. Your discharge is unlikely to be a sign of infection unless it causes itchiness or is foul smelling and greeny-yellow in colour. If you have these symptoms, see your doctor. Many treatments are safe to use in pregnancy, but you'll need advice.

If you suspect you have thrush (candidiasis), always tell your pharmacist that you're pregnant before buying an over-the-counter treatment. Some are unsafe to use in pregnancy.

Self-help for vaginal discharge includes the following remedies:

- Soak a cotton sanitary pad in an infusion of marigold, sweet violet and golden seal (equal parts diluted one part to 15 parts of water) with one drop of tea-tree oil, and wear next to your skin for two hours at a time.

THRUSH

Oral treatment for thrush is becoming an increasingly popular alternative to traditional creams and pessaries. But, according to recent research, nearly half of women buying the over-the-counter medicine have not been asked by their pharmacist whether they may be pregnant. Hormonal changes in early pregnancy make you 10–20 times more likely to get thrush. But the active ingredient fluconazole in oral treatments is not safe to take in pregnancy. Part of the oral treatment's attraction is due to the fact that it's a one-off dose. A safe alternative for women who may be pregnant is Canesten Once cream, a single-dose internal treatment. However, you should always consult your doctor first before using any medicine in pregnancy.

- Avoid sugar in your diet as it increases yeasty fungal growth.

- Increase the friendly flora in your gut by eating live yogurts or drinking lactobacillus drinks. *Lactobacillus acidophilus* supplements are safe to take in pregnancy.

- The homoeopathic remedies Calcarea Carbonica, Sepia and Sulphur are also very useful.

- After 16 weeks of pregnancy it's safe to use a mixture of bergamot, geranium and lavender oils in your bath water. Add two drops of each to 30ml carrier oil (e.g. sweet almond) or milk and throw into your bath water just before you get in.

Weight gain

Normal weight gain in pregnancy is 11–13kg (24–28lb) and includes the weight of the baby, placenta, amniotic fluid and your own body changes. If you start the pregnancy underweight expect to gain 12–16kg (26–35lb). If you're overweight, expect to gain 7–10kg (15–22lb).

WARNING SIGNS TO WATCH OUT FOR

Always ask your doctor for advice on any of the following symptoms:

- vaginal bleeding

- pain on urinating, which could be a sign of infection needing treatment

- severe abdominal pain

- fluid from the vagina that could be leakage of your 'waters'

- change of baby movement – especially lack of it

- high fever (over 38°C or 100.6°F) or chills

- severe vomiting

- blurred vision

- severely swollen face or fingers

- severe headache

- any injury or accident, such as a fall or car crash, which you fear could have harmed the baby

- breast lumps

- a pain in the leg, especially when squeezing the calf or walking, which could be a sign of deep vein thrombosis

- dizziness that could be linked to high blood pressure or anaemia

- excessive itchiness, especially of the limbs.

You started this trimester counting your way towards the middle of your pregnancy. As you complete it, past the halfway mark, look forward to the final phase: preparing for your baby's arrival.

4

THE THIRD TRIMESTER

The final trimester of your pregnancy is the time to think about the remedies and preparations you would like to have at hand for labour and delivery.

By the third trimester, your baby is fully formed but is growing bigger and stronger, ready for birth. By 30 weeks the baby is about 40cm (15$\frac{1}{2}$in) from head to bottom, and by 32 weeks it's likely to be lying head downwards. The skin, which was quite wrinkled before, is now smoother, and both the vernix and lanugo are beginning to disappear.

Around the end of the seventh month, fat begins to deposit on the foetus. It may suck its thumb, hiccup and cry, and taste sweet and sour. It responds to stimuli such as pain, light and sound.

Some time before the birth the baby's head may move down into the pelvis – and is said to be 'engaged'. But sometimes the baby's head does not engage until labour beings.

SYMPTOMS AND SOLUTIONS

Abdominal pain

As ever, you should take serious note of any unusual abdominal pain. But lower abdominal pain may be a symptom of your ligaments stretching to support your growing uterus. Mention it to your midwife or doctor, just to be sure. If it's a continuous problem, or very bad, you could wear a maternity belt, which is designed to give your bump extra support. You can also avoid pain by supporting your abdomen with your hands when you get up from sitting down or lying.

The homoeopathic remedy Bellis Perennis is useful for ligament pain.

Braxton Hicks contractions

From very early in the pregnancy (as early as eight weeks) the uterus begins making practice contractions – but they become more apparent as the pregnancy progresses, and can be quite strong by the third trimester. Early in the trimester, they should not be too painful or regular. True contractions, heralding the start of labour, are regular, intensifying and similar in sensation to period cramps. This kind of pain is always a reason to contact your doctor or midwife.

Women who've already been through one pregnancy are likely to feel Braxton Hicks earlier, and more intensely, than first-time mums.

As the EDD (estimated date of delivery) draws near, your Braxton Hicks may be more frequent, intense and even painful. To relieve any discomfort, change position – get up and walk around, or lie down.

Try a very gentle abdominal massage – stroking your bump slowly and steadily in a clockwise circular motion with one or two drops each of rose, chamomile and lavender essential oils in a carrier such as sweet almond.

Breasts 'leaking'

Your breasts start to produce colostrum, early breast milk, from the second trimester. Some women find this begins to leak – and this is entirely normal – while others have no obvious signs of milk production until after the baby is born. Leave your breasts alone instead of trying to squeeze the colostrum out, and wear breast pads if it's becoming an embarrassing problem.

Breech baby

About 3 per cent of babies are breech presentation – lying bottom down rather than head down at term. And although this used to mean an automatic Caesarean section, many mothers of breech babies do now successfully deliver vaginally. But consider this very carefully before making a decision – and think about the fact that you may still need an emergency Caesarean if the vaginal delivery doesn't proceed successfully.

Prior to 34 weeks there's no need to worry about your baby's breech presentation as it has ample room to turn round and many babies do. But, if towards the end of your pregnancy your baby seems to be sticking to a bottom first position, there are some steps you can take to help the baby turn head-down.

Postural tilting

Lie on the floor with a couple of cushions under your bottom, your knees bent and your feet flat. Remain like this for at least ten minutes. This position creates a little more room in the uterus and your baby may be tempted to turn around.

Acupuncture

The Freedom Fields Hospital in Plymouth had a 60–65 per cent success rate using acupuncture to turn a baby around, but you need a qualified acupuncturist for this. Some acupuncturists found that moxibustion (see page 111) to the acupoint Bladder 67 at the corner of the little toenail can help to turn the baby. It is thought that this helps by increasing the number of foetal movements so the baby somersaults around to the correct head-down position.

Homoeopathy

One dose of Pulsatilla 30c, every two hours for up to six doses (in one day only, then stopped) is recommended. Discuss it with a homoeopathic doctor before attempting this remedy.

Bleeding or spotting

As ever, any bleeding or spotting in the last trimester is bound to concern you. How much of a concern it should be depends on the type of bleeding and the circumstances that surround it.

- Pinkish-stained or red-streaked mucus soon after intercourse or vaginal examination, or brownish spotting within 48 hours, is most likely to be caused by bruising to your sensitive cervix. Report it to your doctor, but it's unlikely to be a danger sign – although you may be advised to abstain from intercourse until after the birth.

YOUR BABY'S PRESENTATION

Breech (see page 56)

Cephalic
Your baby is head-down with the top of the head (the vertex) pointing towards the cervix, and its chin tucked into its chest. This is the best position for delivery as the narrowest part of the head is coming out first and the baby's face is protected.

Anterior
In this position, the baby's back is facing out, lying inside the curve of the mother's abdomen.

Brow
Brow presentation means that although the baby is head-down, the neck is extended so that the brow or face is pointing to the cervix. If your baby is in this position in labour, you'll be closely monitored as the face is less robust than the top of the head. There may also be some facial bruising and/or elongation of the baby's head – but this will quickly subside.

Face
If the baby's face presents first the delivery can be quite awkward and may lead to a delay in the second stage of labour. It's quite a stressful experience for the baby and, as the neck can be flexed backwards in the process, you may want to take your baby to a cranial osteopath in his early weeks of life.

Occipito-anterior or posterior
Occipito-anterior means the back of your baby's head is facing the front of your pelvis as it comes down the birth canal. Occipito-posterior means the back of your baby's head is lying against the back of your pelvis. During delivery the baby's head will probably rotate into an occipito-anterior position, but if it remains occipito-posterior your progress through labour may be slower and more painful – this is known as a 'back labour'. It's demanding for both of you and again may be a good reason to seek out the help of a cranial osteopath while your baby's still tiny.

Transverse lie
This describes the baby who's lying across the womb rather than head-down. If this is the case at the beginning of the labour, a Caesarean section is unavoidable. Transverse lie occurs in one in 250 births.

Unstable lie
A baby is said to have an 'unstable lie' if it keeps changing position between antenatal visits after 36 weeks. Ideally it should be adopting a head-down position around this time, even if the head isn't engaged. If you'd planned a home birth you may have to reconsider going to hospital as a Caesarean section may be necessary.

- Bright red bleeding or persistent spotting could be coming from the placenta and must be checked immediately by your doctor. If your doctor can't be reached, go to hospital.

- Pinkish or brownish-tinged or blood mucus, accompanied by contractions, could be the first sign of labour. Call your doctor or midwife.

Take the homoeopathic remedy Arnica 6c every three to four hours from the moment bleeding starts. This can help hasten recovery and minimise bruising from labour. Other remedies can also be used, depending on the nature of the bleeding – but do consult a practitioner first.

Changes in foetal movements

Babies are at their most active between weeks 24 and 28, but these movements are often erratic and brief, and although always visible on ultrasound, you may not have been aware of them. In the third trimester foetal activity becomes more organised and consistent, with clearly defined periods of rest and activity – especially between weeks 28 and 32.

Comparing baby movements with other pregnant women is always a bad idea. Just like newborns, foetuses have their own individual patterns of development. Some are always active; others tend to be quiet. What matters is that there's no drastic change – for instance where a previously lively baby becomes much slower or even stops moving.

Some obstetricians recommend testing for foetal movements twice a day – once in the morning, when activity tends to be sparser, and once in the evening, when many babies are active.

To check your baby's movements:

- note the time when you start
- count any movements – kicks, flutters or rolls
- stop counting when you reach ten
- often you'll feel ten movements in ten minutes, but sometimes it will take longer
- if you haven't felt ten movements by the end of an hour, take a break, have a snack, then try again.

Changes in the ninth month may be more marked than before. For instance, your baby may seem to squirm instead of kicking. This is most likely to be because there's much less space for gymnastics than there was a few months ago. And, especially when the baby's head is engaged, it will be less mobile. At this stage the fact that you experience regular foetal movement is more important than the type of movement the baby makes.

Continue with tests for foetal movement, as above, because inactivity can be a sign of foetal distress. As long as you're getting your ten movements per test session, things should be going OK. If you don't, contact your doctor at once - picking up foetal distress early through movement testing can prevent potentially serious consequences.

Constipation

If you're just beginning to suffer now, and haven't taken steps to improve your diet, now's a good time to start, as this will also get you in the habit of eating a friendly diet after your baby's born - when constipation can be extremely painful, especially if you've had stitches. See Chapter 2, pages 26-7.

Cord prolapse

The umbilical cord is the baby's lifeline, but occasionally it can slip down into the vagina when your waters break. If this happens the baby's life may be put in danger, so it's important to get to hospital as soon as you can. There a saline solution may be injected into your bladder to cushion the cord, or a cord that's hanging outside the vagina may be tucked back in and held in place by a special sterile tampon and you'll be given drugs to stop the labour while you're prepared for an emergency Caesarean.

Fatigue

This is also likely to increase in the last trimester, for the following reasons:

- you're carrying around more weight than before
- your bulk may be preventing you from sleeping properly
- you may be losing sleep through worry too
- getting ready to have the baby (making work arrangements, childcare plans etc.) can also be exhausting
- you may still be anaemic - especially if you have not been on iron tablets.

As ever, though, fatigue is a sign that you should look after yourself. Rest and relax as much as you can, and save your strength for your delivery.

If you feel no better after resting, report this to your doctor at your next check-up. Anaemia sometimes strikes in the third trimester and some doctors routinely check for it in the seventh month.

For fatigue during the last four to six weeks of pregnancy, drink raspberry leaf tea twice a day, and take 20–30 drops of squaw vine twice daily. Both are considered an excellent preparation for birth. Queen Bee Royal Jelly is also recommended as an energy booster in pregnancy, and is easily obtained in capsule form.

False labour and pre-labour

Nobody knows exactly what triggers labour. But prostaglandins, natural substances made by the body, are thought to play an important part in the process. These are produced by the uterus during pregnancy and increase during spontaneous labour. They stimulate uterine muscle activity and trigger oxytocin release by the pituitary gland, both of which help to move the labour along. But prostaglandins alone are not responsible for labour and a combination of foetal, placental and maternal factors are responsible for setting labour in motion.

Pre-labour symptoms, which can start a full month before the real thing (or sometimes only an hour before) include:

- engagement of the baby, two to four weeks before labour in first-time mothers, but often only just before labour with later births

- crampiness in the pelvis and rectum

- persistent low backache

- slower weight gain

- change in energy levels – for better or for worse (we don't all get the nesting instinct that makes some pregnant women spring-clean their houses just before giving birth)

- thicker vaginal discharge

- 'show' – a pink or bloody discharge as the cervix effaces and dilates, rupturing capillaries. If this happens, labour is very close

- loss of mucous plug – a gelatinous chunk of mucus (which has sealed the cervix and has now come loose because the cervix is beginning to thin and open for labour) is sometimes passed through the vagina a week or two before the first real contractions, but this may not happen until just before labour begins

- more intense Braxton Hicks contractions

- diarrhoea.

False labour symptoms include:

- irregular contractions that are not increasing in frequency or severity

- pain in the lower abdomen, rather than the lower back

- contractions that are relieved by walking around

- foetal movements that intensify briefly with contractions – though be aware of excessive foetal activity, which could be a sign that the baby's distressed.

Premature labour

Labour that begins before the 37th week is premature. But only 7–10 per cent of babies are premature, and most of these are born to women who are already known to be at high risk.

Factors predisposing a women to premature labour include:

- smoking

- alcohol

- drug abuse

- poor weight gain – if you were significantly underweight before getting pregnant you should aim to gain around 35lb (just under 16kg) in pregnancy

- poor nutrition – see the guidelines on page 11

- standing for long periods every day

- sexual intercourse (only if you're already at high risk)

- hormonal imbalance

- infections – early labour may be the body's way of getting the baby out of a dangerous environment. For this reason, stay away from people who are ill, look after your own nutrition and use a condom for intercourse later in pregnancy
- a weak or incompetent cervix
- irritable uterus – this can set off untimely contractions. If the problem is diagnosed, bed rest should help delay labour
- placenta praevia – a low-lying placenta
- chronic maternal illness – high blood pressure, heart, liver or kidney disease, or diabetes
- stress
- age under 17
- age over 35
- structural abnormalities of the uterus
- multiple pregnancy
- foetal abnormality
- history of premature babies.

Occasionally none of these risk factors is present, so it is important to take notice of the following symptoms of premature labour – however well things have been going thus far. Symptoms to look out for are menstrual-like cramps, lower back pain or a change in the nature of lower backache, achiness in the pelvic floor, thighs or groin, a change in your vaginal discharge (especially if it is watery or bloody) or broken waters – a trickle or a rush of fluid from your vagina.

Treatment

Prompt medical attention is vital to postpone premature labour and give the baby a stronger chance of survival (unless there are very good reasons why the baby would be better off being nurtured outside the womb). If you have strong contractions but no bleeding, you may simply be admitted to hospital for supervised bed rest. If the membranes are intact and the cervix has not dilated, there's a good chance of carrying your baby to term.

Oedema

Oedema is swelling due to the accumulation of fluids in the tissues. Some degree of swelling is considered completely normal – 75 per cent of women experience it, and especially towards the end of the day, in hot weather, or if they've been standing for a long time. Usually it disappears overnight though.

You can help relieve the discomfort of oedema by putting your legs up, wearing comfortable shoes and avoiding elastic-top socks or stockings. Support tights can also help – but put them on first thing in the morning, before the swelling has started.

Keep on drinking plenty of water (2 litres a day). This helps prevent water retention, but don't drink it all at once. Two glasses at a time is sufficient. Reflexology is good for reducing the swelling caused by fluid retention in pregnancy. Taking vitamin B6 (10mg daily) has been shown to prevent oedema and may reduce it if taken once it has become a problem.

(NB If your hands or face become puffy, notify your doctor as this could be the first indication of pre-eclampsia and will need speedy treatment.)

Overdue baby

It's distressing to think your baby is 'late'. The phone never stops ringing with anxious friends and relatives wanting to know how you are, and this can add to your own stress. But studies show that, in spite of our efforts to pin down the right EDD, 70 per cent of apparently late babies are not late at all. They are only believed to be late because of a miscalculation of the time of conception.

If you reach 42 weeks, your doctor will check the size of the uterus and the height of fundus (the top of the uterus), and match these against the timing of the first foetal movements you felt and the first heartbeats detected by your midwife or ultrasound technician. The doctor will then want to be sure that the baby is continuing to grow and thrive well into the tenth month, but, even if it is, conditions in the uterus will begin to deteriorate as time goes by. The placenta is getting on a bit, and can no longer provide adequate nutrition and oxygen, and the production of amniotic fluid also drops. This can make things difficult for the baby and babies who are born after spending a long time in these less than perfect surroundings are called 'post-mature'. They are thin, with dry, flaky skin, and none of the vernix coating that most newborns have.

They may also have long nails, thick hair and alert, open eyes. Those who have been in the post-term uterus the longest may be yellow stained and at greatest risk during labour, or even before labour. Because of their size, they're likely to have a difficult delivery and may even have to spend some time in the special care baby unit.

For these reasons, if your doctor wants to induce the labour, it is unwise to think about resisting.

Overheating

Your body is naturally warmer during pregnancy – so dress sensibly in layers of cotton clothing to allow your skin to breathe. Take frequent baths and continue to drink plenty of cool water.

Pubic pain

Pubic pain is not unusual in the last two months as the cartilage between the two sides of the pelvis softens to allow the pelvis to move more freely in childbirth. Massaging the area with rosewood or lavender oil mixed with a carrier oil (such as sweet almond) may help. If the pain continues, you must report it to your midwife or doctor.

Sexual worries

A lot of women are confused about the advisability of having sex towards the end of the pregnancy. But many doctors and midwives allow women with healthy, uncomplicated pregnancies to continue making love right up to their EDD. And most couples manage this without any problems. However, if you're in a high risk category for premature labour, intercourse may start you off early. If this could relate to you, talk to your doctor about the best course of action.

Sex is also sometimes linked to infection antenatally and postnatally. So a condom should be worn in the last eight weeks of pregnancy. Whatever your worries, don't be afraid to discuss them with your doctor or midwife.

Skin problems

The PUPPP (pruritic urticarial papules and plaques of pregnancy) lesions, which sometimes gather in stretch marks and on the thighs, buttocks and arms, aren't dangerous to you or your baby – and will disappear after delivery.

Stretch marks

Stretch marks across the growing abdomen and breasts are caused by the skin stretching so quickly that its collagen fibres become damaged. If well oiled, however, the skin will remain supple throughout pregnancy – and stretch marks can be avoided.

Make sure your diet is rich in vitamin E, and rub vitamin E oil into any emerging red marks. Wheatgerm oil, scented with a drop of lavender oil, also works wonders.

Stress incontinence

As the baby's weight and pressure of the growing womb push down on your bladder, stress incontinence may become more of a problem. There's not much you can do to prevent it now – but keep up your pelvic floor exercises to prevent post-natal incontinence.

Vulval soreness

Soreness can indicate infection, so it's important to check this out with your doctor before taking any steps to remedy it yourself. But washing the area with lavender water, then swabbing with a dot of tea-tree, rosewood or geranium oil blended in a base of jojoba can help.

Remember that all the care you've given yourself during these nine months will have put you in tune with your body in preparation for the birth. As you come to the end of your pregnancy, be confident in your ability to deliver a healthy baby.

5

LABOUR AND BIRTH

You've looked after your diet, learned to relax, and done your exercises. What more can you do to prepare your body for childbirth?

PREPARING FOR CHILDBIRTH

Drinking raspberry leaf tea is recommended to tone the uterus for labour and birth. One teaspoon of tea infused in a cup of boiling water, up to three times a day, is the suggested dosage. Raspberry leaf is what herbalists call a 'partus preparator'. It is the best known of a group of herbs used in preparation for childbirth. Others include lady's mantle, red clover, St John's wort, blessed thistle, hawthorn, motherwort, goat's rue, nettle and fennel. Native American Indian women also use squaw vine, blue cohosh, black cohosh, birth root, cramp bark and false unicorn root. Self-Heal Herbs make a Pre-Natal Formula which is to be taken in the last six weeks of pregnancy only.

Raspberry leaf tea tones and strengthens the uterus, making it more flexible for labour. However, it should only be used in the last trimester of pregnancy, as it has been known to overstimulate the uterus. If you do find that your Braxton Hicks contractions are increasing, cut back on the dosage.

Massaging the perineum (the area between the pubic bone and the coccyx, which takes in the urethra, vagina and anus) can be started two months before the expected birth. It is a good way to increase suppleness in preparation for labour and birth. Massage the area daily with wheatgerm or almond oil, or calendula (see page 146).

PAIN RELIEF – PLANNING AHEAD

For some women labour is short and straightforward, and the level of pain is quite manageable. For others, it's a long and difficult process, and the pain is beyond a level they can cope with. If you approach labour feeling confident and well informed, with an open mind about the kind of pain relief you may need, you stand the best chance of a happy experience.

The uterus uses a lot of energy, which it makes from glucose and oxygen in the bloodstream. Strong contractions can cut down the blood supply and energy to the uterus muscle, and products such as lactic acid can build up, causing contractions to feel more painful.

If you have kept fit during your pregnancy, this will give you more flexibility and stamina in labour. Remaining upright and mobile during contractions will also help.

As labour builds up, your body produces endorphins, which are natural pain relievers that are also produced during exercise. These act on the brain like an anaesthetic, reducing the sensation and perception of pain. However, they are rarely enough to see you through labour without additional pain-relief, be it self-help, or a complementary or orthodox remedy.

Natural pain relief

Breathing

Breathing exercises have been taught at antenatal classes for years and are one of the most basic, but effective, ways of dealing with pain. During your preparation for childbirth, practise breathing out slowly and deeply with your partner. In labour, deep, slow breathing will help you cope with contractions. A partner who understands the routine can help you slow down if you start to panic breathe (which can cause hyperventilation and dizziness).

Distraction

Keeping yourself busy, as far as possible, will take your mind off the early stage of labour. When labour is well established, singing or listening to favourite music can help. Visualising yourself in a special place can also work wonders. Get to know, in advance, what works best for you.

Hot and cold compresses

A cold compress (a wrung-out towel or an ice pack) can help pain in the lower back. You may find warm towels or flannels on your perineum, or a hot water bottle on your lower back, are comforting and relaxing.

Massage

Having your scalp, shoulders, arms and lower back massaged by your partner can be comforting in labour. Practise in advance, so your partner knows what you like. If you're new to massage, the basic rules are to keep warm, and use oil or talc to soothe bare skin. Your partner should use a firm, steady pressure and emphasise each downward stroke.

Relaxation

Relaxation exercises learned during pregnancy and practised in labour will enable oxygen to flow to your muscles, cutting down on muscle tension and making contractions less painful.

Water

Sitting on a stool or chair under the shower can feel wonderfully relaxing, especially if you direct the jet towards the part of you that's hurting most. Many hospitals have large baths you can soak in once your cervix is dilated beyond 4–5cm, and a birthing pool, if you have access to one, is fantastic for pain relief – even if you don't plan to give birth in it.

Complementary therapies

If you want complementary medicine for childbirth, explore all your options early on, and always seek the advice of an experienced practitioner.

- Acupuncture triggers the release of endorphins, the body's natural painkillers. The points that are stimulated are the uterus, shenmen and endocrine, which target the relevant area, provide general pain relief to the whole body, and help stimulate contractions. A few hospitals have midwives trained in acupuncture.

  Others use TENS (transcutaneous electrical nerve stimulation) machines as a substitute, as the lower electrodes cover key acupoints. TENS relieve pain via four electrode pads on your back which discharge electrical currents. The idea is that these currents block the pain you would otherwise be experiencing. The method takes some getting used to, and should be practised from early pregnancy if you're planning to use it. It has no known ill-effects on the baby, but the main drawback is that, for some women, the method is totally ineffectual!

- Acupressure is a useful alternative to acupuncture if you do not have access to a practitioner. Your birthing partner can use the balls of his or her thumbs to apply weight to the acupoint Bladder 23 (see page 113 for location). This weight should be steadily and evenly increased as you breathe in, then held for about five seconds, and released again as you breathe out. You can practise this before going into labour.

- Aromatherapy is great – as long as you're not one of those women who hate being touched once contractions start. The combination of essential oils and massage are an excellent way to ease back pain and relax you generally, but you will need a willing partner or midwife to massage you. The Active Birth Centre makes a labour oil containing geranium, marjoram, clary sage and lavender.

- Bach Flower Remedies may also relax you and lift your mood. They may be useful combined with other forms of pain relief.

- Homoeopathy stimulates the body to heal itself and may help relax you. Specific remedy suggestions are listed below.

- Hypnotherapy has been shown by researchers to be more effective in relieving pain than some of the strongest drugs, including pethidine. It involves visualisation, which allows you to mentally 'turn down' the intensity of the pain, like turning down the heat of the cooker. Some women can even switch off the pain completely. A good hypnotherapist should be able to write you an individual programme during pregnancy, which will be automatically triggered once labour starts. However, not everybody is good at self-hypnosis and you may find it difficult to concentrate.

- Reflexology can improve your breathing and induce deep relaxation. Hold your hand out with your fingers gently curved towards you. Your partner should apply gentle thumb pressure to the dip in your palm just below the fleshy pad beneath your middle finger. The pressure should be applied in time with your in-breaths and released with your out-breaths. Massaging around the crease of the joint at the base of your thumb on each hand will help to calm your mood and ease tension around your shoulders and neck.

LABOUR – RECOGNISING THE REAL THING

In Chapter 4 the symptoms of false labour and pre-labour were outlined. Once the contractions of pre-labour are replaced by stronger, more painful, and more frequent ones, the labour is probably for real if:

- the contractions intensify and aren't relieved by a change of position
- they become progressively more frequent and painful
- you have a pink or blood-tinged 'show'
- your waters break.

If you're in any doubt, call your doctor or midwife and, in any case, call them if you know you're in labour. They'll tell you what to do next. Don't be put off by a fear of embarrassment in case it's not labour, and don't delay too long unless you're planning a home birth, everything is ready, and your midwife lives extremely close by. Even though the start of labour may herald a long wait ahead, it is an unpredictable process and you must be prepared for a short labour too.

Early labour (up to 4cm dilated)

The cervix at the bottom of the womb has softened and ripened during pre-labour. Now it's starting to open. As it does so, the mucous plug inside the cervix comes away – you experience this as a pink or bloody 'show'. Sometimes labour begins with a sudden breaking of your waters, or a slow trickle.

Try to stay relaxed now – it will help the delivery. Eat high-energy foods such as pasta, bananas, toast and honey, but check with your midwife as labour progresses that it's OK for you to continue eating and drinking.

Drink chamomile tea to calm you and quench your thirst.

Active labour (4 to 10cm dilated)

As your uterus contracts to pull the cervix open over the baby's head, it also moves forward to push your baby down hard on to the cervix where the pressure of the baby's head helps the cervix to open.

The more relaxed you are, the better your uterus will work.

Active labour lasts an average of two to three-and-a-half hours – but variations on this average are wide. The uterus can achieve more in less time, with contractions becoming stronger, longer and more frequent (3 to 4 minutes apart and lasting 40 to 60 seconds). Each contraction should have a distinct peak – but they may not be as regular as you'd expected.

Stay as upright as you can and lean forwards, never backwards. Kneel forwards on the floor or on the bed, over a beanbag or a pile of pilllows. Or lean into your partner's arms. The all-fours position is very popular and allows you to rock from side to side during a contraction. Your partner can also reach your back easily if you want it stroked or massaged.

Now's the time to focus on your breathing to stop yourself tensing against the pain. Breathe out through your mouth; many women find sighing or groaning deeply helps a lot.

Stretch whichever part of your body you find yourself tensing. If your hands are clenched in tight fists, stretch out your fingers and sigh out through your mouth at the same time. If you can't remember to do this during a contraction, take the opportunity in the space before the next one comes along.

Choose from the following herbs for the first stage of labour:

- raspberry leaf and squaw vine infusion (30g to $^1/_2$litre of water for each herb). The squaw vine helps to open the dilating cervix, while the raspberry leaf facilitates contractions. If you don't want to drink teas and infusions, use four drops of the tincture of each herb
- cramp bark or back haw for painful contractions
- valerian tincture as a painkiller
- tincture of Californian poppy, skullcap or motherwort to calm you.

Transition (preparing to push)

You've reached the end of the first stage of labour when you feel an irresistible urge to push down. Transition is the end of this stage, when the intensity of contractions picks up with peaks that last almost the 60–90 second duration of the contraction. Some women experience multiple peaks and you may feel as if the contractions never completely disappear.

You are likely to have a lot of pressure in your lower back or rectum and may feel as if you want to open your bowels. You may be grunting involuntarily and your body temperature may change, making you warm and sweaty or chilly and shivery. More capillaries in the cervix will rupture, increasing your bloody vaginal show, and you are probably exhausted. When you reach this stage, your midwife will give you a vaginal examination to check that you're almost 10cm dilated. As soon as you are, you will be allowed to start pushing.

If your midwife says you're not ready to start pushing, pant or blow instead. Try chanting out loud, 'Hoo, hoo, ha!'. Pushing against a cervix that isn't completely dilated can cause it to swell, delaying delivery.

Pushing

Now, when you have a contraction, the baby is being squeezed by your uterus down the elastic tunnel of your vagina, between the bony passage of your pelvis.

With luck, you will get a second wind for this stage of labour.

Get into a pushing position. Semi-sitting or squatting is best because gravity will be on your side to give you more pushing power.

The more effectively you push, the more quickly the baby will get through the birth canal, so listen carefully to your midwife's instructions and when you hear, 'Push!', give it your all! If you're too frantic or disorganised in your pushing you will waste energy and achieve little.

Birth

Your baby's head will stretch the skin of your perineum and emerge, followed by the shoulders and the rest of the body. This may take several contractions but the midwife's hands will be near to ensure that your baby comes out safely. If you're able to stay on all fours for the delivery, your baby's head will stretch the tissues at the back of the vagina more gently and you're less likely to tear. If you need an epi-siotomy, this will most likely be caused at the height of a contraction – when the pressure of the baby's head numbs the area.

The umbilical cord will be cut and clamped at once, and your baby will be handed to you for a cuddle and you may feel a surge of love for her… But don't worry if you don't. For many women the main feeling now is overwhelming relief that labour is over.

Use aromatherapy oils applied locally to relax or stimulate you. One or two drops each of chamomile, rose and lavender in 50ml of almond oil can be used for a firm lower back massage to help relax you. Or apply a cold compress of lavender and rose geranium to your forehead or wrists.

Delivering the placenta

Many hospitals routinely administer an injection of syntometrine into the mother's thigh as the baby emerges. This makes the uterus start contracting again to deliver the placenta and minimises bleeding. Take a deep breath and bear down when asked, to help the placenta slide out.

COMPLICATIONS AND VARIATIONS

Back labour

So called 'back labour' means the baby has the back of his head pressing against your sacrum. This is very painful and the pain often doesn't let up between contractions.

- Try changing your position to take the pressure off your back. Crouch or squat to get on all fours to make yourself more comfortable. If you don't feel up to moving, or have to stay in bed because you've been given pethidine or you're attached to monitors, try to lie on your side with your back well rounded.
- Press a hot water bottle or even an ice pack against the area to soothe the pain.
- Acupuncture can help too – apply strong finger pressure to just below the centre of the ball of your foot.

Caesarean section

A Caesarean section may be recommended early in your pregnancy because of some foreseen complication, in which case you will be given a date and will know exactly when you are having your baby. An emergency Caesarean takes place when a problem is identified during labour. The operation can be performed under general anaesthetic or epidural. The epidural has the advantage that you can see your baby as soon as she has been pulled out, and this is very important for some women who feel they are missing out on the birth if they are unconscious. Some doctors, recognising the strong desire in women physically to push their babies out, will ask you to give a push as they lift the baby out. You can expect the following during a Caesarean birth:

- your pubic hair may be shaved

- you'll have a catheter inserted into your bladder to keep it empty

- if you're to be awake for the operation (i.e. you're having an epidural anaesthetic), a screen will be put up at shoulder level so you won't see the incision being made

- sterile drapes are arranged around your exposed abdomen and the area is washed down with antiseptic solution

- an IV (intravenous) drip is set up so that additional medication can be given if it's needed

- in an emergency Caesarean, things may move very quickly

- your partner may be asked to leave the room, depending on the hospital's policy

- if you are awake, you may feel the incision as a sensation of being unzipped – but you should feel no pain

- a first cut is made in the lower abdomen before a second incision, in the lower segment of your uterus

- the amniotic sac is opened and any remaining fluid is suctioned out. The baby is then eased out, manually, or with forceps, and you may feel some tugging

- at this stage, if you want, the screen can be lowered slightly so you can see the baby being delivered, but are spared the gory details

- the baby's nose and mouth are then suctioned and you'll hear her first cry before the cord is clamped

- you may be given syntometrine intravenously to help your uterus to contract and any bleeding to be controlled

- don't be alarmed if your baby is whisked away. Babies born by Caesarean section often need resuscitation after the birth because they have not had the benefits of a vaginal birth to stimulate their own respiratory system.

(For recovery from a Caesarean, see Chapter 6.)

Episiotomy

An episiotomy is a small cut in the perineum to enlarge the vaginal entrance just before the baby is born. The procedure used to be performed routinely by many hospitals, but there's now a growing movement against it.

In its favour, the episiotomy is thought to prevent serious tearing, make stitching more straightforward, and prevent prolapse in later life.

Against the procedure, midwives claim that small tears mend and heal better, and with less discomfort, than an episiotomy, many episiotomies extend into ragged tears anyway and some even increase the risk of later prolapse.

However, in special circumstances, an episiotomy may still be required, often alongside forceps, as follows.

- Your baby may be in distress, in which case she will need to be delivered quickly. Forceps will protect her head so she's not subjected to pressure during the birth – and an episiotomy is almost invariably used alongside forceps.
- You may be too exhausted to push – or an epidural may have rendered pushing impossible.
- You may have high blood pressure and be advised not to push too much.

If you have an episiotomy – or a tear – it should be sewn up as soon as possible after the baby's born, with plenty of local anaesthetic. The layers of the vagina, the muscles of the perineum and the skin all have to be closed separately – but usually with thread that dissolves rather than having to be taken out.

Make a warm water spray with calendula tincture to apply to the area to make it more comfortable. Arnica cream around the stitch line will ease bruising. You can also take the homoeopathic remedy Arnica 6c three to four times daily. Bathe the area in warm water containing three drops each of cypress and lavender oils – or more if your skin will tolerate it.

Forceps or ventouse

Forceps may be required in the following circumstances:

- to turn the baby's head if the presenting part is too wide to descend through the birth canal

● if you're too tired to push hard enough to finish delivery without help

● your baby's distressed

● there's a delay in the second stage of labour.

Any doctor making a decision to use forceps should keep you fully informed about why the procedure is necessary in your particular case. When forceps are used, you'll be given a local anaesthetic before the curved blunt blades are cradled one at a time around the baby's temples so it can be gently delivered.

Ventouse or vacuum extraction is a popular alternative to forceps and involves suctioning the baby out of the birth canal with a cap applied to its head. It has the advantage that it can be used before the cervix is fully dilated – whereas forceps require full dilation of the cervix.

If you have concerns about the possible use of forceps or ventouse, discuss them with your midwife before you go into labour.

To avoid bruising, follow the advice given for episiotomy, especially arnica.

Forceps babies may be fractious and twitchy, in which case you can give them the Bach Flower Remedies Star of Bethlehem (for trauma) and walnut (to adjust to change), or the homoeopathic remedies Arnica 6c or Kali Phosphoricum 6c – one drop on the tongue twice daily.

Induction

Most inductions take place because the pregnancy has continued past term, and the placenta is beginning to deteriorate. In mothers over 35, placental insufficiency is more common after 40 weeks, so induction may be recommended earlier for older mothers than for younger women (who may be allowed to go to 42 weeks).

Other reasons for induction include high blood pressure, a labour that hasn't progressed more than 24 hours after your waters have broken, a weak or erratic labour, or prevention of a potentially difficult labour and delivery if you've previously had a large baby.

Your labour may be induced in one of the following ways, depending on the method of choice of your obstetrician:

● Prostaglandin pessaries may be administered to ripen the cervix enough to start labour off.

20 WAYS TO GET YOUR LABOUR GOING

1. **Get active.** When your baby is due – or overdue – a daily walk and even a bit of dancing around the house will encourage it to engage, which in turn will encourage labour to begin.

2. **Drink raspberry tea leaf** – but not too much of it (about three cups a day).

3. **Eat curry.** Spicy foods are great if your baby is overdue. They have a similar (though not so fierce) effect to old-fashioned castor-oil, stimulating the bowels, which in turn will help trigger the start of labour – though nobody knows exactly why.

4. **Make love.** Semen contains natural prostaglandin. In hospital you'd probably be given synthetic prostaglandin in pessary form to induce labour.

5. **Practise yoga** during the early stages of labour. Sitting with the soles of your feet together and knees flopping out ('tailor' position) will allow the pelvic area to relax.

6. **Use gravity.** In early labour, being upright and moving around as much as possible will help things along by encouraging the baby's head down, exerting more pressure on the cervix. Walking or moving during a contraction can help you cope with the pain, while squatting on a small stool between contractions opens the pelvis. When you're upright the uterus is tilted forward, and there's no weight bearing down on the major blood vessels, so you have a better flow of blood and oxygen to the baby enabling it to stay in good condition throughout labour. Your sacrum is also more mobile and this means the pelvis joints can expand and adjust to the shape of the baby's descending head.

7. **Dim the lights.** The psychological benefits of soft lighting and a cosy environment are often underestimated. But your body needs to feel safe, secure and relaxed before the birth hormones can really get going so labour can progress unhindered.

8. **Get in water.** It doesn't have to be a birthing pool – a warm bath, or even a shower, will do. Water encourages the flow of hormones, as well as feeling good and being relaxing.

9. **Be with someone who cares.** The support of a birthing partner – be it your midwife, husband, mum or best friend – is vital. Trials have consistently shown that having someone there 'for you' can reduce the need for pain relief – and it can even prevent an unplanned Caesarean. In Canada and the US, women hire professional birthing partners called Doulas – Doula is a Greek word which means an experienced woman who helps other women. The practice is now starting to take off in the UK, too, and, over the next few years, Doulas may become quite commonplace. The Doula (or birth companion or labour assistant) will be knowledgeable in childbirth and helps provide continuous physical and emotional support throughout the latter stages of pregnancy and labour.

10. **Write a birth plan.** You can even state: 'I want the emotional support of my midwife.' Hospitals do read these plans and take them seriously, and, if you're happy and comfortable with the way your labour is being managed, you'll be more relaxed, and things are more likely to move on smoothly.

11. **Have your nipples stimulated!** Be alone with your partner for a bit. Stroking or massaging the nipples helps trigger the release of the hormone oxytocin, which helps move labour along. In trials nipple stimulation has been proved more effective than syntocinon, the synthetic hormone administered by injection to induce contractions.

12. **Switch off from the pain.** If you're in pain, you're more likely to be frightened and tense, and will find it difficult to let your body open up. Hypnotherapy and visualisation will help you manage the pain (see page 70).

13. **Use herbal medicines.** Four drops each of tincture of squaw vine (to open the dilating cervix) and raspberry leaf (to encourage contractions) in a teaspoon of water.

14. **Use your sense of smell.** In labour, the aromatherapy oil, clary sage, comes into its own. You should avoid using it throughout pregnancy because it is so powerful it can stimulate contractions – but during labour it is ideal. Put a few drops in an aromatherapy oil burner, or in a bowl of hot water, or even on a hot flannel that you sniff. If you feel like being massaged – and not everyone does – add a couple of drops to the massage oil.

15. **Make the most of homoeopathy.** The remedy Caullophyllum is ideal if you need to encourage more productive contractions, for example if they've so far been weak, or you've been dilating very slowly. But you will need to consult a homoeopath during your pregnancy if you want this remedy.

16. **Get to know your body's acupoints.** Reflexologists and acupuncturists both use a point on the heel of the foot to stimulate labour. They avoid touching this area in pregnancy, because it's known to be so effective in producing contractions – but get a practitioner to mark the point for you so that your partner can put it to use in the delivery room.

17. **Tune into your breathing.** Don't worry about specific breathing techniques – they're far too complicated when you're in labour. Instead, just focus on your out-breath, following it through to the very end. Your in-breath will take care of itself. Focusing on your breath will keep you in the moment, rather than worrying about what's happened or what's still to come.

18. **Make a noise.** Sing or blow raspberries. Making a noise is helpful – but it's got to be positive noise. Screaming and squealing will only tense your body up, but singing or making sounds with your out-breath will keep your mouth open and relaxed, and this has a direct effect on the vagina and pelvic area. You can test the theory for yourself by clenching your teeth and trying to relax your pelvic floor at the same time. It's impossible to do it. But if you try to relax your pelvic floor while blowing raspberries or singing, you'll find it much easier.

19. **Don't push before you're ready.** If you think you are fully dilated – but your midwife is telling you you're not – pant or blow yourself. Pushing against a cervix that isn't completely dilated can cause it to swell, delaying delivery.

20. **Don't panic.** If things slow down at the end of the first stage, and you're fully dilated but have no desire to push, this is your body's way of saying it's really exhausted and needs a short break before summoning up the energy it needs for you to give birth to your baby. If you can just relax for 10 to 20 minutes and wait for the urge to push, then you can work with your body for a more productive second (pushing) stage, instead of trying to struggle on when you're too tired.

- Your waters may be broken, as the sudden loss of amniotic fluid can bring the baby's head down and this in itself can stimulate labour.

- You may be given an injection of syntocinon (a synthetic hormone) to stimulate contractions.

- If your baby's overdue and you want to help it on its way, you can try to induce labour by making love – semen contains small amounts of prostaglandins, which help to soften the cervix. Having your nipples stimulated may release the hormone prolactin, which also softens the cervix.

- Acupuncture does help bring on labour – but can take several treatments over three or four days. An acupuncturist may put in tiny semi-permanent needles that allow you to apply pressure to the point yourself.

- Cranial osteopathy can help by stimulating your pituitary gland – though it takes a couple of days to work.

- Goldenseal can help contractions to become more regular. Take 2.5ml of the tincture every hour with something sweet to counter the bitter taste.

Long labour

Your labour will progress well with strong uterine contractions that open the cervix, and a baby who can fit your pelvis. If the contractions are too weak, or your baby is too large (or your pelvis too tight), then you may be in for a long labour. It is considered a long labour if there's little or no dilation after 20 hours, if you're a first-time mum, or 14 hours if this is not your first child. Sometimes the delay is because the contractions you've felt are those of a false labour, but there's also a theory that some women panic at the onset of labour, triggering the release of chemicals in the nervous system that interfere with contractions.

If contractions stop for about two hours during active labour, there's a 50:50 chance it's because of a disproportion between the size of the pelvis and the baby's head. But the labour may slow down due to plain exhaustion.

The baby may move very slowly down the birth canal (at a rate of less than 1cm per hour in women having their first babies), but the birth may be otherwise uneventful. You may have your waters broken, or be administered oxytocin, to speed things up.

If the pushing stage lasts longer than two hours, your doctor may want to use forceps or perform a Caesarean. But if steady, though slow, progress is being made, and both you and your baby are doing well, the natural vaginal delivery will be allowed to go ahead, possibly with gentle easing of the head with forceps. Staying in a squatting or semi-sitting position at this time will help with the delivery.

- The homoeopathic remedy Pulsatilla 6c helps regulate contractions. Gelsemium 6c is useful if they're slowing down and tiring you. Take either one every two or three hours.

- Use a fingernail to dig into the acupoint beside your little toenail to stimulate contractions.

- A bath with a few drops of clary sage will also help labour along.

- Korean ginseng, ginger drops or capsules, and Bach Rescue Remedy help if labour is long and you are exhausted.

Twins or more

Many twin pregnancies remain uncomplicated right through childbirth, with a normal vaginal delivery. However, there are still some obstetricians who believe all multiple pregnancies should be delivered by Caesarean section. And there is definitely more potential for complications during the delivery of twins – so even if a vaginal delivery is scheduled to go ahead, an anaesthetist will be on hand in case a Caesarean is needed.

The most likely complication will arise from the babies' positions in the womb during labour. When both babies are head first, a vaginal delivery may be attempted. But one baby may be delivered vaginally and then the other will move and become unturnable, requiring a Caesarean section. So be prepared for the unexpected!

Water birth

Using a birth pool is no longer considered an 'alternative' practice. Many hospitals encourage women to use water – for labour if not delivery – as it helps reduce pain. According to Sheila Kitzinger, who has campaigned to give women the choice of water birth, half of all women who use water in labour go on to give birth in the pool, too. And she reports that they often believe that the water provides a more gentle transition to life for the baby, who has been floating in amniotic fluid for nine months.

8 THINGS THAT WILL INCREASE YOUR PAIN
– AND TIPS TO HELP YOU COPE

1. **Fatigue** Take plenty of rest during your ninth month.
2. **Expecting pain** Try to distract yourself.
3. **Being alone** Make sure you have a birth partner lined up.
4. **Being hungry or thirsty** Have light snacks during early labour, and sip water throughout.
5. **Stress or anxiety** Remember your relaxation and breathing exercises.
6. **Fear** Read up about childbirth before the event so you know what to expect.
7. **Feeling sorry for yourself** Concentrate on the reward at the end.
8. **Lack of control** Educating yourself about childbirth will give you more confidence to cope with the event.

However, critics of water birth argue that there may be an increased risk of problems such as infection for both mother and baby, trauma to the baby, perineal trauma and post-partum haemorrhage.

If you are considering a water birth, speak to an organisation such as the Active Birth Centre, who can put you in touch with a midwife who's familiar with water deliveries and the safety guidelines for using birthing pools.

Water birthing pools hold 100 gallons of water (weighing 450kg) – so, if you're planning to have a pool at home, make sure your floor can stand the weight, and that your water tank holds enough water to fill it (most domestic tanks hold a maximum of 70 gallons).

Many hospitals have birthing pools. These are not used routinely – though you may be considered for a water birth in hospital if:

- you have had a problem and risk-free pregnancy, and no potential complications have been identified

- your baby's size is compatible with your ability to deliver safely

- you're at least 38 weeks pregnant when you go into labour

- your baby is head-down, not breach or transverse

- there's no sign that your baby's distressed and your baby's heart has been monitored and found to be satisfactory.

If you've read this chapter prior to going into labour, try not to dwell on what can go wrong, but what can go right! The majority of deliveries are straightforward – and by remaining as calm as possible as you go into labour you will enhance your enjoyment of the birth.

6

POST-PARTUM

Although your pregnancy has ended with the birth of your baby, the first six weeks after the birth are a crucial time for your recovery. You may feel you want to concentrate all your attention on your new baby's needs, but your own health remains just as important.

It's natural for a new mum to spend all her time on the new baby, but it is also very important to look after yourself. Don't be afraid to ask for help with the daily chores of shopping, ironing and so on. Get other people involved. You might even get your partner to take some unpaid leave from work. Don't be afraid to catnap during the day when the baby is asleep. This helps to recharge your batteries and boost your energy levels. If you do have any worries or concerns, such as feeling low, or just tired, there are many people who can help you. Contact your health visitor, midwife or doctor for advice. No matter how trivial the problem may seem they will be happy to advise you and give you any help they can.

YOUR PHYSICAL RECOVERY

Afterpains

Afterpains or strong contractions of the uterus are particularly likely to be experienced when the baby is feeding, but are more common with second, third or fourth babies than the first one. These pains are a result of the uterus returning to its normal size.

Herbal anti-spasmodic drops are a very useful remedy to help the uterus contract to its pre-pregnancy position and to relieve pain. They can be brought ready-made from suppliers and you should take 10 to 20 drops in water just before breastfeeding, as the baby's sucking causes contractions. If you can't find the ready-made drops, try black cohosh or cramp bark, both available in tablet form.

Breastfeeding

Today's paediatricians and midwives will encourage you as far as possible to try breastfeeding. And even if you can only stick it for a couple of weeks, your baby will have benefited. There are many advantages of breast over bottle:

- Convenience: breast milk is there whenever you need it. There's no need to fiddle around preparing bottles.

- Antibodies: the colostrum prepared by your breasts during pregnancy becomes the baby's first feed and is full of antibodies that protect your baby from the diseases you've had and have been immunised against, as well as safeguarding them from the bacteria that causes gastroenteritis. Bottle-fed babies are more likely to get gastroenteritis, and if you have chosen to bottle feed, or are supplementing breast with bottle, it is vital that you make sure the teats of the bottles are properly sterilised.

- Breast milk provides everything the baby needs. For the first four months of your baby's life, all the drink and food he needs can be obtained from your breast milk. Your breasts have the amazing ability to manufacture according to the seasons too, so that in hot weather your milk will quench his extra thirst without compromising on the food aspect of his feed.

- Breast milk protects your baby from allergies, infections and often obesity.

- Your baby's nappies are not as smelly as those of babies being fed on formula.

- It is cheaper than buying formula and bottles.

- It is more restful for you than feeding with a bottle.

- It provides closeness, which aids the bonding process between you and your baby.

Contrary to popular myth, the size of your breasts has nothing to do with the amount of milk you make. Milk production is controlled by the hormones prolactin (responsible for quantity) and oxytocin (which delivers the milk through the nipples to your baby).

Oxytocin causes the milk-producing cells to contract, squeezing the milk down the ducts and out of the nipple. This is known as the let-down reflex – and is sometimes so efficient that your breasts feel as if they are full enough to burst, making the baby's feed time very welcome when it comes.

Sometimes the let-down reflex makes milk drip from one breast while you are feeding the baby with the other. If you want, you can catch this milk and freeze it for later use, or even donate it to a Special Care Baby Unit.

Positioning the baby correctly is important. Make sure you are comfortable too – you could be stuck in this position for some time!

Your baby should be facing you sufficiently centrally so that he has to tilt his head back to get your nipple in his mouth. When he is correctly positioned you can see the muscles at his temple moving as he feeds. If his cheeks are going in and out he is not on properly and you will have to put your little finger into the corner of his mouth, take him off, and start again.

The first few feeds of your baby's life are provided by the colostrum your breasts have produced during pregnancy. This is a transitional feed from placental feeding to milk, and is gentle on your baby's new digestive system. After a few days the colostrum is replaced with breast milk which provides two types of milk – foremilk and hindmilk. The foremilk is low in fat and calories and satisfies the baby's thirst. The hindmilk is the richer milk that gives the baby his meal.

Breastfeeding problems

Blocked ducts cause a tender lump and can make you feel feverish. This can follow engorgement (see overleaf) or pressure on the ducts – maybe because your bra is too tight, or you are feeding your baby in an awkward position. Even if you're tempted to stop feeding, don't – it will make things much worse. Instead, try to massage the lump gently in the direction of the nipple to clear the blockage, apply hot and cold compresses, and offer that breast first at frequent feeds so that the baby's strongest sucking (at the beginning of the feed) will help get the milk moving through the ducts again.

- Make a compress for your breast by soaking a breast pad in one drop each of rose, geranium and lavender oils diluted in 500ml cold water.

- Use garlic capsules, vitamin C and echinacea tincture (15 drops in a glass of water) to fight infection.
- Homoeopathic remedies will treat specific descriptions of the condition. Aconite, Bryonia, Calcarea Carbonica and Belladonna are all helpful. If the breast seems to be getting infected, take Mercurius.

Engorgement can cause your breasts to become hot, swollen and hard, and is caused by the increased blood flow to the breasts.

- Cold compresses applied to your breasts will help bring the swelling down, and washing your breasts in warm water before a feed will help the milk to flow more quickly, which will also help.
- Mix three drops of geranium oil into a non-allergenic cream and massage over the breast.
- Applying a bruised cabbage leaf to your breast (leave it inside your bra and replace as necessary for up to 24 hours) has a guaranteed anti-inflammatory effect.
- Take echinacea tincture (15 drops in a glass of water) to prevent infection.

Insufficient milk may be due to stress, an inadequate diet, or not enough rest on your part.

- An infusion of any of the following herbs – dill, fennel, caraway or aniseed (1–2g per cup) – helps to encourage milk production and will also prevent your baby from developing colic.
- Tincture of borage (starflower) or evening primrose oil will provide the essential fatty acids needed to build up your milk supply.
- If your milk supply has failed completely, take chaste berry in a tincture or tablet form for up to one month.
- Acupuncture and acupressure may help release more milk. The point to work on is Small intestine 1 (see page 113).

Sore or cracked nipples are most common in the first week or so as you adjust to breastfeeding. You can help prevent this by expressing a few drops of hindmilk at the end of each feed and smoothing it over the nipple and areola.

- Apply a little marigold (calendula) or chamomile ointment after each feed.

- Use undiluted witch-hazel – but remember to wash it off before your baby's next feed.

- Expose your breasts to the air as much as possible.

- If the nipples are sore, cracked and blistered, and feel worse at night, use the homoeopathic remedy Graphites. If the pain spreads all over the body during feeding, take Phytolacca. For simple soreness, take Calendula internally, while also applying the tincture externally.

Mastitis can cause similar symptoms to a blocked duct and may be non-infective, caused by milk leaking from the blocked duct and surrounding tissue. Infective mastitis also has the same symptoms – but you may feel more ill. The infection may be caused by a germ in your baby's nose that is transmitted to your breast. Follow the same guidelines as for treating engorgement (page 86) and blocked ducts (pages 85–6), and see your doctor about antibiotics (but remember to mention that the antibiotic needs to be suitable while you are breastfeeding). If tests show that your milk is infected, you may have to stop feeding temporarily from the affected breast. Your midwife or health visitor will be able to give you advice about the best way to go about this.

Bruising

Your vagina has been stretched and the muscles worked hard during labour, and you will naturally feel sore and bruised as a result.

Soak a sanitary pad in diluted tincture of calendula, witch-hazel or St John's wort, freeze it and then wear it next to your skin until it thaws out.

Caesarean recovery

After a Caesarean, your body has to recover from two major traumas – childbirth and surgery. Be gentle on yourself. You need plenty of help – especially in the first week, when you shouldn't do any lifting or housework. If you must lift the baby, lift from waist level, using your arms but not your abdomen. If you have to bend, use your knees, not your waist.

Many women worry that their stitches will burst if they move too much, but there is no danger of this – even though at first you need to support them to avoid pain when you cough, sneeze or laugh. The stitches will come out around the fifth day, but, while they're still in, you can wear high-waisted pants and a press-on sanitary towel (for your lochia blood loss) to avoid rubbing them.

Your scar will remain sore for a few weeks, but will slowly improve. During this time it's normal to feel brief pains around the scar – and these are part of the healing process. These pains may be followed by a period of itchiness from the scar, which is also quite normal. However, persistent pain, redness or discharge are all possible signs of infection – so see your doctor if you experience these.

- After a Caesarean, take the homoeopathic remedies Arnica and Calendula for several days. If the Caesarean was unplanned and against your wishes, take Staphsagria.
- Use acupuncture to treat a scar that remains painful or does not heal well.

Clots

It is normal to pass clots of blood after the birth – but, if you do, you should try to retain the clot to show it to your midwife who will be able to check that it is indeed a clot and not a piece of retained placenta (see pages 90-1).

Coccyx pain

The coccyx (tailbone) is pushed backwards at the baby passes through the birth canal. If it feels painful afterwards, take St John's wort. Although best known as an antidepressant, herbalists also recommend it for chronic nerve pains and for trauma and injury involving nerve damage. If the problem lasts longer than a few days, an osteopath should be able to relieve it.

Constipation

You lose a lot of fluid in the first few days after giving birth and consequently many women find they are constipated. You'll want to avoid constipation as far as possible, as straining on an already delicate and stretched area is extremely uncomfortable, so drink plenty of water and make sure your diet is rich in fibre – wholegrains, fruit and vegetables. Laxatives are better avoided as they can be passed through your breast milk to your baby.

- Fybogel, which you can buy over the counter to bulk out your food, will not affect your baby.

- Osteopathy can help if the problem becomes long-term. This can be more likely after forceps.

Fluid loss

During pregnancy your body will have stored up excess fluid, which is now shed in the first few days after delivery. You need to empty your bladder frequently and may sweat heavily too. You are also bleeding from the vagina, and beginning to produce milk from your breasts. All in all, you may feel like a leaky sieve. Take showers to help yourself feel more comfortable, and drink plenty of water to help combat constipation. Losing fluid is normal – but do tell a doctor if you are feeling unwell with it.

Lochia

Lochia is the name given to the vaginal bleeding you experience after childbirth. For the first 48 hours it is likely to be quite heavy – much heavier than any period you have experienced – you will probably need to use large maternity pads. The midwives checking you will let you know if the loss is too heavy or is cause for concern. After the first two days the blood loss lessens, but altogether it will continue for anything from two to six weeks after the birth.

You can control excessive lochia by applying pressure to a point just in front of the webbing between the big toe and the one next to it on the upper side of your right foot.

Post-partum haemorrhage

Bleeding after the delivery of the baby can threaten the mother's life if not stemmed quickly. Thankfully, due to drugs now available to help the uterus contract and thus stop bleeding, it is rarely a fatal condition these days.

Causes of post-partum haemorrhage include the following:

- A uterus which, even after a normal delivery, does not contract satisfactorily, allowing bleeding to continue. An injection of ergometrine or syntometrine (syntocinon with ergometrine), often combined with gentle massage, will help the relaxed uterus contract into a tight ball, at which point, bleeding should stop. If the uterus fails to relax, it's most likely to be because it's exhausted after a prolonged labour or because of overdistension by a multiple birth. If in excess of 2 litres of blood is lost, this is a sign of polyhydramnios – a potentially dangerous condition which occurs in about 3 per cent of pregnancies.

- Retained placenta (see below).

- Occasionally a very large fibroid may hinder uterine contractions and this makes haemorrhage more likely. Repeated injections with ergometrine or syntocinon should quell bleeding.

- A large tear in the cervix, maybe because of a rapid or forceful labour, or a very large baby, can cause quite severe bleeding. But the cervix can be repaired with stitching and this will stop the bleeding.

- Infection can cause a haemorrhage right after delivery, or weeks later.

- Having had placenta praevia or abruptio placenta prior to delivery makes post-partum haemorrhage more likely.

- Rarely the cause is a previously undiagnosed bleeding disorder that interferes with the blood's ability to clot.

The symptom of post-partum haemorrhage is any abnormal bleeding after delivery. This means any bleeding that saturates more than one pad an hour for a few hours or is bright red any time after the fourth post-partum day – especially if it doesn't slow down when you rest. Foul-smelling lochia, large blood clots, pain and swelling in the early days after delivery also need to be reported to your midwife.

In the worst scenario, a blood transfusion will be needed to replace blood lost during the haemorrhage.

Homoeopaths recommend taking Arnica and Kali Phosphoricum at birth to prevent haemorrhage.

Retained placenta

Usually the placenta separates and is delivered spontaneously a few minutes after delivery of the baby. In about 1 per cent of all deliveries, the placenta will not separate, and this is called a retained placenta. Its presence in the uterus prevents the uterus from contracting after the birth, and this increases the risk of a haemorrhage – so removing it becomes a matter of urgency. This can be done manually, or by a D&C (dilatation and curettage, which scrapes out the contents of the womb). But, very occasionally, if the placenta has grown into the wall of the uterus a hysterectomy may be the only option.

- A massage with jasmine oil aids placental separation.
- The homoeopathic remedies Caulophyllum 6c and Pulsatilla 6c every one to two hours until separation may work – although not instantly.
- Acupuncture and cranial osteopathy can help too, but you would need to have a practitioner on hand very quickly for these to be realistic options.

Stitches

If you have had stitches, for either a tear or episiotomy, you will feel quite uncomfortable for a few days. The scar will feel enormous and swollen – but rest assured your perineum will return to normal in a few weeks.

Soothing remedies such as homoeopathic Arnica or tincture of Hyper-Cal (which you can put on a pad) help speed up the healing process and reduce soreness.

Stress incontinence

Stress incontinence can start after childbirth, when the pelvic floor muscles are weakened and 'leaking' becomes a problem – especially when you laugh, cough or sneeze. It is embarrassing to live with – and difficult to discuss. But doctors are very used to treating incontinence – so do not be put off making an appointment to talk through the problem. In most cases treatment will be very straightforward.

Before going to the doctor, ask yourself the following questions – and keep a note of your answers.

- Do you 'leak' when you laugh, cough or sneeze, or when you move suddenly or bend to lift something?
- Do you have a constant, intermittent dribble?
- Do you often not reach the toilet in time?
- How often do you go to the loo?
- Once you have the urge to go, how long can you hold on?

- Does your bladder empty without warning?

- Do you wet yourself at night?

- If so, does your wetting wake you – or are you unaware of it until morning?

- Has your flow of urine changed – is it not as good as it once was?

- Do you often feel thirsty?

- Are you taking any drugs? If so, which ones?

Your doctor will need the answers to these questions (and there may be others too) for clues about what is causing your incontinence. You may also be asked to keep a chart showing how much you have eaten and drunk in a day, and how often you have passed urine, and tests may be ordered to further establish or rule out the cause of your incontinence.

The tests will determine whether you have diabetes or an infection or if your incontinence is a response to medicine you are taking.

You may be referred to an incontinence adviser and a gynaecologist and physiotherapist. Drug therapy can also be prescribed to help recapture and maintain continence. Your continence adviser, if you're referred to one, will help you make the best of the healthcare available – getting the right appliances, garments, bedding and care that you need. A physiotherapist will give you exercises to do to strengthen your muscles. You may also be offered electrical stimulation, e.g. interferential therapy, which makes muscles relax and contract. This treatment is given in an outpatient department, but there is an alternative, functional electrical stimulation, which you can be trained to use at home.

- Make sure you keep doing the exercises you are given, and that you work at any bladder retraining you are given.

- Use vaginal weights, available from your continence adviser, to increase vaginal tone.

- Keep charts to monitor your progress.

- Try to get your bladder completely empty every time you go to the loo – pressing a tissue firmly against yourself and waiting a few seconds to encourage those last drops to come.

- Use your district nurse and continence adviser – they're there to help you, so don't be afraid to ask them for help.

- Wear clothes that are simple to remove, and nothing that is too tight around the stomach or bladder where it can increase the pressure to go to the loo.

- At night go to the loo before getting ready for bed, and then again just before going off to sleep so your bladder is quite empty.

- If late night drinks make a difference, take your last drink earlier in the evening – and keep a drink by your beside in case you're thirsty in the night. If you do have a drink in the night, go to the loo before going back to sleep.

- Naturopaths recommend cutting out caffeine, which acts as a diuretic, and cutting down on artificial sweeteners, carbonated drinks and tomato-based foods, which can all irritate the bladder.

- Gingko can help to tone the urinary system.

- Biofeedback (see Part Three, Chapter 28) can be used to help you identify and strengthen the relevant muscles for better bladder control.

- The homoeopathic remedy Causticum 6c is recommended for involuntary urination after sneezing, coughing or laughing.

Uterine inversion

Very rarely, when the placenta doesn't detach completely after the delivery of a baby, it pulls the top of the uterus with it, like pulling a sock inside out. This is uterine inversion and causes excessive bleeding and shock.

You are at slightly increased risk of this happening if:

- you've had many babies

- you've had a prolonged labour (more than 24 hours)

- the placenta is implanted across the top of the uterus

- you were given magnesium sulphate in labour (sometimes used in the treatment of pre-eclampsia)

- the uterus is overly relaxed or the fundus isn't firmly held in place while the placenta is coaxed out in the third stage of labour.

Usually the uterus can be replaced by hand – though occasionally surgery is necessary. If there's been a lot of blood loss, you may need transfusions.

Venous thrombosis

Sometimes, in the pregnant mother's body's efforts to prevent a bleed, the opposite happens, and the blood over-clots. It's natural for the blood's clotting ability to increase in pregnancy, but, combined with the enlarged uterus, which can make it difficult for blood in the lower body to return to the heart, this poses an increased risk of venous thrombosis – a blood clot that develops in a vein.

Clots in superficial veins (thrombophlebitis) occur in about one or two in every hundred pregnancies. Deep vein thrombosis, which if untreated can result in the clot moving to the lungs, thus threatening the patient's life, is much less common.

You are slightly more at risk of developing a clot if:

- you're over 30
- you've had three or more previous deliveries
- you've been confined to bed for long periods
- you're overweight, anaemic or have varicose veins
- you've had a forceps or Caesarean delivery

In superficial thrombophlebitis there's usually a tender, reddened area that runs in a line over a vein that is near the surface in the thigh or calf. In deep vein thrombosis, the leg may feel heavy or painful, there may be tenderness in the calf or thigh, swelling, distension of the superficial veins, and calf pain when you flex your toes towards your chin.

With deep vein thrombosis an anticoagulant drug (e.g. heparin) is usually given intravenously for about a week to ten days, then under the skin until labour starts, at which point treatment is stopped until several hours after delivery, when it's resumed and continued for a few weeks.

EMOTIONAL PROBLEMS

The baby blues

You may have a couple of days of feeling sad and rather weepy – usually coinciding with your milk coming in. About half of all mothers suffer with the blues. They may last for a few hours or, at the most, for a few days, and then they disappear.

The symptoms – feeling very emotional and upset – may seem irrational. You can't tell what brought your tears on, but nothing you try will clear them up either! Some mothers feel very anxious and tense, and minor problems may be blown out of all proportion.

The cause is the change in hormone levels you experience after delivering your baby. Throughout pregnancy hormone levels rise to accommodate the baby and, by the time labour begins, levels of progesterone and oestrogen are 50 times higher than they were before the pregnancy. After the birth, these levels fall suddenly and dramatically so that within hours they are below the levels they were at before the pregnancy began.

Mothers who have the blues should be allowed the freedom to cry and to express their fluctuating emotions. If they feel miserable they should not be told to pull themselves together, but instead listened to, and reassured that the misery will soon pass. A mother with the blues is very sensitive to anything medical staff and friends and relatives may say – so tact and empathy are key words for carers at this time.

Surprisingly little information about postnatal depression (PND) is given to expectant mothers. Yet 10 per cent of recently delivered mums go on to develop this sad illness. And although some will actually need psychiatric help and drug therapy, it is important to note that all cases of PND do eventually pass – and you need not be separated from your baby during your illness and recovery.

But the taboo that still surrounds PND puts many women off speaking up about their fears that they may be postnatally depressed. And this can make matters worse, because, of course, they are not getting the support they need – and, in effect, have to suffer in silence.

So, how can you recognise the symptoms, and deal with them?

If your baby blues seem to be getting worse, and the symptoms are becoming more distressing, depression could be developing – although for some women the baby blues pass and then, several weeks after the birth, depression starts to set in. But, in fact, it is not always easy to recognise that you are depressed because, since the baby's arrival everything has changed – and it is easy to blame your symptoms on all the new demands on your time and energy.

However, it is possible you are suffering from some degree of depression if you notice several of the following symptoms:

- you feel permanently tired and lethargic
- simple household chores seem too much effort
- you can't be bothered to bathe, dress properly or care for your appearance
- you suffer from head, neck or back pain
- you feel generally unwell
- you are anxious – worrying unjustifiably about the baby and other members of the family
- you can't cope with meeting friends or even answering the door
- you experience confusion or panic in an everyday situation
- you can't relax, no matter how much you know you should
- you develop obsessional thoughts
- you can't concentrate on books, television programmes or even conversation
- you sleep badly
- you lose all interest in sex.

Sometimes the care of a small baby is too much to cope with and you should not be afraid to ask for help from a relative, friend or neighbour while you recover. Ideally you will want someone to come in to your house and help with the domestic chores, giving you time to rest. Being separated from your baby is likely to exacerbate your depression – and it is unlikely anyone will suggest this when an alternative can easily be found.

If you think you may be suffering from postnatal depression you should see your doctor. Your local health visitor will also be able to help.

Your doctor may prescribe tranquillisers or antidepressants. They may make you feel drowsy – but this usually wears off as you continue to take the drug.

If you find that the drugs make you feel worse in any way, consult your doctor to see if you need a stronger or milder dose, or a different form of treatment.

Although using antidepressants can seem quite frightening, these drugs have an important role to play in 'buying' time for your recovery. They can make the unpleasant symptoms fade until they go completely.

Severe cases of postnatal depression may require a stay in hospital while you recover. There are now several special mother and baby units where depressed mothers can receive the treatment they need, while keeping their babies with them. Your doctor will be able to tell you where these are and to help you get into one if this is viable for you.

During your recovery you can help yourself a lot by believing in your ability to get better. But you need patience and you have to understand that recovery will take time.

Take as much rest as you can. This is important because tiredness seems to make depression worse. If you can, try and rest on your bed (sleeping if possible) every day. Avoid late nights and try to get someone else to feed the baby if possible. Some doctors believe that rest, peace and quiet, after the birth can help to prevent postnatal depression – so rest must play an important part in your convalescence.

Try not to go without food for long periods as hypoglycaemia – low blood sugar – can make things worse for a depressed mother. If you're trying to diet, cut down on sweet, starchy foods and eat plenty of fruit or raw vegetables when you're hungry.

Finding small chores you can easily complete will help occupy you as soon as you are ready for this – and will take away those feelings of uselessness that come with having nothing to do when you are depressed. This is sometimes known as 'polish your shoes' advice – but, done slowly and steadily, simple tasks can help restore order to your life, as well as being quite therapeutic.

For many women with feelings of postnatal depression, there is nothing more helpful than talking their problems through with someone who's been through the same thing and who really understands how they feel. Support groups exist especially for mothers who have been postnatally depressed (see Useful Addresses) – and the women you'll meet there will have had a range of experiences, some of which may make you feel you aren't doing so badly after all, and others will jolt you into understanding that, yes, you do have a problem that deserves all the time and care you can lavish on yourself.

Puerperal psychosis is the name given to a mental illness (such as manic depression), which manifests itself for the first time postnatally. It is not caused by childbirth, but happens because you are already predisposed (as are one in four of the population) to mental illness, and the pregnancy, birth or postnatal period put you under the strain that triggers an attack.

There is nothing specific about pregnancy or childbirth that provokes mental illness. In most cases, any other emotional disturbance of similar severity would equally act as a trigger.

- Cranial osteopaths believe that postnatal depression is caused by the downward displacement of the uterus following the birth and the resultant tug on the pituitary gland via the dura (a continuous thin membrane that lines the brain and spinal cord). Some cranial osteopaths claim they can help postnatal depression in just two weeks.

- Acupuncture has a good record for treating depression.

- Homoeopathic treatment throughout pregnancy may prevent postnatal depression. If it does develop, however, Natrum Muriaticum 6c taken three times daily is a classic remedy.

- Medical herbalist Carol Rogers recommends the following combination of herbs to treat postnatal depression: tinctures of chaste berry, St John's wort, borage and oats used in equal parts and taken in a 5ml dose three times a day. Borage (starflower) oil is specifically recommended for postnatal depression and can be taken in 500mg capsules three to four times a day in addition to your postnatal formula.

- The essential oils of jasmine, clary sage and ylang-ylang are also recommended for postnatal depression. Mix in equal parts and add one drop to your bath water, or evaporate one drop in an essential oil burner.

Remember, problems are not an obligatory part of your first three months with your baby. This is also a precious time when you get to know your new child – so forget the washing up and ironing if you can, and enjoy!

Part Two

Complementary Medicine for Children

7

GENERAL TIPS ON CHILD HEALTH

The ailments of children under five covered in this chapter are all minor and will usually resolve themselves in time. However, there are plenty of things parents can do to help their child become more comfortable and even speed up the healing process. Inevitably, on some occasions your child will not improve or may get worse and will have to see a doctor. It is not always easy for parents to know when their child is truly ill and many feel that they will be bothering the doctor unnecessarily. This is understandable but rest assured that most doctors feel the best judge of a child's health is the parent.

So if you feel your child is unwell and needs medical attention be confident in your own observations and speak to your doctor who can either give advice over the telephone or suggest that it would be best to see your child at the surgery. Many parents worry about taking a sick child to a surgery and often insist on a home visit. These fears are unfounded. The best place for an ill child is the surgery, where the child can be seen quickly and the doctor has everything at hand to make a thorough examination and, if required, do certain tests.

Babies and toddlers cannot tell you they are ill, so you have to rely on your intuition, and certain clues and signs. Some of the most important are as follows:

- A usually active child starts moping and becomes uninterested in her toys.
- A child who previously slept and ate well but now is constantly irritable, difficult to feed and console.
- Constant crying in a baby.

- Continued diarrhoea and vomiting, combined with a refusal to eat or drink.

- Dry nappies for over 9–12 hours.

- Rashes. Most are caused by reaction to a minor viral illness such as a cold. A few rashes are due to infectious diseases such as chickenpox and rubella. Most rashes are self-limiting and just need time to disappear by themselves. Most rashes will fade if you put pressure on them with a finger or a glass. The colour then comes back as you take your finger off or lift the glass. This is called 'blanching'. If the rash does not blanch it needs to be seen by a doctor straight away. It can sometimes be caused by meningitis.

Finally even if your child has none of these signs but you feel something is wrong – speak to your doctor who will be happy to help.

FOOD AND DRINK

Adults lose their appetite when they are ill and children are no different. Children should never be force-fed but food should be presented to them often so they can snack. Fluids are particularly important to avoid dehydration and these should be actively encouraged. Giving your child her favourite food and drinks will encourage them to eat and drink more. Do not worry if your child loses weight – she will quickly put it back on as soon as she recovers.

Sometimes babies will refuse all bottle drinks but are happy to continue breast-feeding. A good way to give them more fluids is to drip water or juice into their mouth with a plastic spoon from a cup. For babies who can bottle feed – again try giving the drink little and often, say, $\frac{1}{2}$oz every 15 minutes.

Rehydration sachets (such as Dioralyte), which contain salts and sugar, are available from the chemist. One sachet per 8oz of water makes a good drink and is often better tolerated by babies, as it is quickly absorbed into the body as soon as it passes into the stomach. Various flavours are available.

Although these techniques can take a long time to administer they are good ways of getting adequate fluids into your baby.

Older children should be advised to sip drinks slowly – just to 'wet the inside of their mouth'. Another good technique – always popular with children – is to give them ice-pops to suck.

FEVER

A high temperature is a reaction to illness and will make your child feel unwell. However, having a slight temperature is not always a bad thing because it helps the body fight the illness. The bugs causing the illness cannot survive much above normal body temperature so trying to get the temperature down to normal is not necessary. But if the temperature is high (above 38°C/101°F) you can bring it down by several methods that often work better together:

- Take off your child's clothes and leave her in just her underwear or nappy.

- Don't cover her up in a quilt or a blanket. If she feels too cold or starts to shiver cover her in a cotton bed sheet.

- Give her plenty of cold drinks.

- Use a fan. Don't point it directly at the child; have it on to cool the room.

- Don't allow the room temperature to get too high – keep it at about 20°C.

- You can open a window in your room to allow in fresh air but don't let your child sit in a draught.

- Try tepid sponging: a damp cloth on the forehead will often suffice. This needs to be regularly soaked in water every few minutes and replaced on the forehead. If the temperature is very high, sponging your child all over in an empty bath with luke-warm water will help.

- Paracetamol is an excellent way of bringing down temperature and is the first thing you should try. It can be given to any child over three months of age and is available from your chemist. It can also be given to children under three months, but speak to a doctor before you give it. Don't exceed the dose on the bottle. The paracetamol will work within 30–45 minutes and many children feel considerably better after taking it. Paracetamol *can* be taken with cough mixtures and antibiotics. It will also help with any aches and pains, such as earache or a sore throat. The first thing your doctor will often ask you is whether you have tried paracetamol.

- Ibuprofen syrup is also available from your chemist. Used instead of paracetamol for fever and pain relief. Do not give to children with asthma.

- Homoeopathy: Aconite 6c (sudden onset of fever, chilly, restless); Nux Vomica 6c (cannot get warm); Pulsatilla 6c (weepy and upset); Belladonna 6c (flushed and restless). All remedies should be taken three to four times daily until the fever settles.

SPECIFIC AILMENTS

Children suffer from many ailments throughout their first few years and it would be impossible to consider them all in this book. However there are some illnesses that most children will suffer from at some time or another and many of these respond well to complementary therapies. These are the ailments that we have considered below. Homoeopathic remedies are available in tablets, powders and drop form. One tablet is approximately the equivalent of three drops. For the homoeopathic remedies below, either give one tablet or three drops to your child as instructed. All the remedies recommended can be taken with conventional treatments such as paracetamol, ibuprofen and antibiotics should your child require these as well.

Bumps and Bruises

- Cold compresses and rest are the best first-line treatment.
- Homoeopathy: Arnica 6c every 15 minutes after the injury until pain is reduced. If there is a sprain (e.g. to the ankle or wrist) try Ruta 6c.
- Herbalism: apply witch-hazel to sprains or a calendula compress for bruises.

Car sickness

- Acupressure: press on the inner forearm about two fingerbreadths above the wrist crease. Gentle pressure should be applied for 1–2 minutes every 15 minutes. If old enough your child can be taught to apply the technique herself.
- Herbalism: eat ginger (biscuits, crystallised or in a drink).
- Homoeopathy: Coccolus 6c or Tabacum 6c – take 30 minutes before the journey.

Colds

These are due to viruses and are usually associated with sore throat, fever, runny nose, headache, earache and cough. Some children can even develop a rash with these viruses. There is no cure for the common cold and antibiotics do not help. Colds usually last seven to ten days and children under five can get six to 12 colds a year. That's almost one a month. This is important, as this is the way your child builds up immunity to the bugs that we all breathe on a daily basis.

- Herbalism: echinacea given three times a day strengthens the immune system. A popular all-purpose tea for colds is made from equal parts of elderflowers, yarrow and peppermint. For children the tea can be sweetened with honey and sipped throughout the day.

- Homoeopathic treatments: Aconite, Natrum Muriaticum, Bryonia or Arsenicum 6c, three times daily for five days.

Colic

- Picking up your baby and carrying her over your shoulder may comfort her and ease the pain. A warm water bottle gently pressed on the tummy can also help.

- Gripe water helps in some cases. The most popular drug for colic in babies is Infacol. Give 0.5–1ml before each feed. The drug makes it easier for the baby to get rid of excessive wind.

- To stop your baby getting colic always wind her well after a feed.

- If a bottle-fed baby has a problem with cow's milk protein (in formula milk) it might help if you switch her to a soya preparation. Try the soya for three months and then reintroduce the formula milk. A few babies need to continue soya milk indefinitely. Breastfed babies can be helped if the mother gives up drinking cow's milk – trying drinking soya, rice or goat's milk instead.

- Herbalism: a weak infusion of fennel or dill given three or four times a day will help. These can be sweetened with honey if required.

- Homoeopathy: Colocynth 6c or Magnesium Phosphoricum 6c four times daily during the attack.

- Aromatherapy: It is not recommended you use essential oils on a child below one year old as their skin is particularly delicate. Instead, a ten-minute gentle body massage with almond oil can help (see Massage in Part Three, Chapter 19). Ideally, the massage should be carried out half-an-hour after a feed.

Conjunctivitis or 'sticky eye'

- Make up some salt water (a *level* teaspoon in a pint of cooled, boiled water) and wipe the eye with it, using cotton wool balls every two hours. Start as soon as you notice the discharge.

- Herbalism: bathing the eye with an infusion of marigold helps, as this herb has good antiseptic properties.

- Homoeopathic remedies: Apis Mellifica, Pulsatilla 6c three times daily for five days. Also try Euphrasia mother tincture – dilute two drops in half a glass of cooled, boiled water and use to wipe the eye.

- Some mothers have found that wiping the affected eye with breast milk can also improve sticky eyes.

Coughs

- Steam inhalation is the most useful way of helping a child's cough. Boil a kettle in your bathroom or toilet so it's almost like a sauna. Then sit in the steam with your child for 20 minutes. Repeat up to three or four times a day. Steam from a hot bath will also help.

- Honey and lemon in hot water will soothe tickly coughs and help to break up any mucus on the chest. Teas from marshmallow will ease an irritating cough, while wild lettuce is a good cough suppressant.

- Herbalism: a herbal chest rub can help loosen phlegm: five drops each of fennel and hyssop essential oils; ten drops each of eucalyptus and thyme essential oils. Mix in 50ml of a base oil (such as sunflower or almond) and massage into the chest two or three times a day in children over a year old. Babies under a year can be helped by putting a few drops of the mixture on a handkerchief and tying this to the foot end of the cot.

- Homoeopathy: Aconite or Belladonna 6c three times daily for five days.

Cradle cap ('baby dandruff')

- Washing with medicated shampoo and then vigorous brushing of the affected area with a soft brush will help.

- You can also rub the area with medicated soap on a wet, rough towel.

- Gently rub in some olive oil into the affected scalp. Leave for two hours, then rub vigorously with a rough, dry towel. Shampoo the excess olive oil away at baby's bathtime.

Diarrhoea and vomiting

See the advice for giving fluid to your child under the 'Food and drink' section above. Also, try the following:

- Homoeopathy: Arsenic Album 6c for diarrhoea. Ipecac. 6c or Nux Vomica 6c for vomiting three times daily for five days.
- Herbalism: Use an infusion of agrimony – three to four cups a day.

Earache

- Homoeopathy: Aconite 6c (if in severe pain); Belladonna 6c (if flushed); Chamomile 6c (if restless and irritable). Take every two to three hours for two days.

Eczema

- Herbalism: Apply marigold ointment three times daily. Warm cabbage leaves applied to the area also stop irritation and soothe inflammation.
- Homoeopathy: Sulphur 6c or Mercurius Sol 6c every two to three hours at times of a severe attack.

Nosebleeds

- Homoeopathy: Arnica 6c or Aconite 3c three times daily.

Sunburn

- Herbalism: Calendula compresses or baths will soothe the skin.
- Homoeopathy: Belladonna 6c (if hot and flushed) or Cantharis 6c (if blistering is present) three times daily for five days.

Teething

- Homoeopathy: Chamomile 6c or Pulsatilla 6c can be applied straight to the gums three to four times daily.

Fortunately most of these conditions are self-limiting and will resolve themselves with time. However, if your child does not improve within a few days or seems to be getting worse do seek medical attention. Remember the best judge of your child's health is you – if you are worried or simply want to put your mind at ease contact your doctor.

Part Three

Complementary Therapies Explained

IMPORTANT NOTE
Always tell your doctor or practitioner that you are or maybe pregnant *before* taking any medicine or undergoing any treatment.

8

ACUPUNCTURE AND ACUPRESSURE

Acupuncture has been around for over five thousand years – and the first book on the subject, written between 475 and 221 BC, is still available. The Chinese came up with the idea after soldiers, wounded by arrows, were mysteriously cured of illnesses in other parts of their bodies.

The therapy is based on the belief that an internal force of energy ('chi') runs through our bodies. It is made up of two opposite forces, 'Yin' and 'Yang', which meet up at the surface of the body in strategic areas (acupoints). An imbalance of chi is thought to cause disease.

WHEN SHOULD YOU TRY ACUPUNCTURE?

Acupuncture can be used to help treat numerous problems in pregnancy – check your symptoms against suitability for treatment in Part One of this book.

The main advantages of acupuncture are that it is safe to use in pregnancy and while breastfeeding; it brings relief of pain unresponsive to conventional therapy and decreased use of painkilling tablets and injections; a feeling of relaxation after therapy; and it works well with all conventional therapy and is easily available.

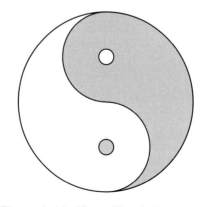

The symbol for Yin and Yang indicates the perfect balance and constant interaction of energies in healthy existence

The acupuncture practised today uses a series of 14 imaginary lines called 'meridians', which each join a group of acupuncture points. Most meridians are named after one of the internal organs. For example, the 'colon' meridian starts at the tip of the index finger, runs up the arm and ends at the side of the nose. Other meridians similarly criss-cross the body. Meridian and acupuncture charts are widely available illustrating the human body and, where the practitioner is a vet, cats, dogs and elephants.

Firm fingertip and thumb pressure on an acupuncture point, or acupressure, will cause a short-lived effect and this is particularly useful to try on yourself at home (see Chapter 27). Shiatsu, Tui Na and Zero Balancing are all forms of acupressure. Practitioners will often use their palms, elbows, knees and feet to apply pressure on chosen points.

Considerable scientific research has been carried out on acupuncture and most researchers now believe that it exerts its effects by releasing natural hormones called endorphins and enkephalins within the body. These then affect parts of the central nervous system, blocking pain and altering control of bodily organs. Acupuncture may also change the way that pain messages are sent to the brain and might even block these messages. Research has also shown that acupuncture can also increase local blood supply and the release of natural steroids and chemicals involved in the sensation of pain.

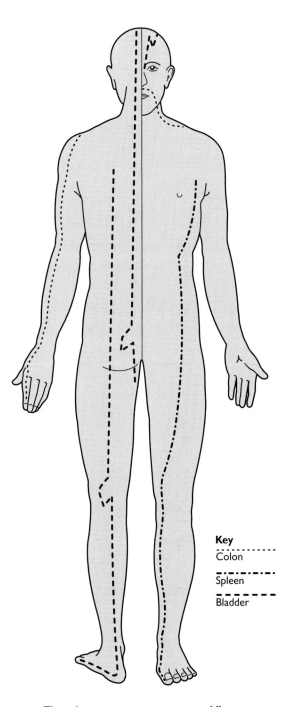

Key

- - - - - - - - -
Colon

- ⋅ - ⋅ - ⋅ -
Spleen

- - - - - - -
Bladder

Three important acupuncture meridians

WHAT CAN YOU EXPECT?

There are over two thousand acupuncture points but modern practitioners often use no more than two hundred of them in their day-to-day practice – and these will be chosen very specifically for your own individual needs. If your condition is suited to acupuncture treatment, and you have a good therapist, you have a 65 to 70 per cent chance of being successfully treated.

The treatment itself involves needles finer than a hypodermic being carefully inserted through your skin and left in for between 10 to 45 minutes (depending on the condition being treated). The number of needles varies but may be only two or three. The skin is stretched and the needles are usually inserted to a depth of between 0.5–2cm, depending on the area of treatment and the patient's build.

Your therapist may use a technique of alternately rotating, withdrawing or pushing the needles in further. To begin with you're likely to need treatment sessions once or twice a week – but it's normal to move on to longer intervals between appointments as your condition responds. Your practitioner might also ask you to return every few months for a 'top-up' session to keep the problem at bay.

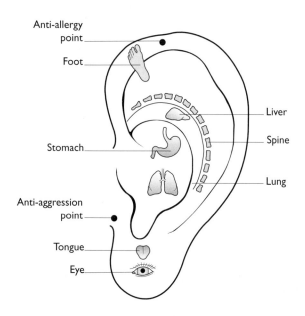

Ear acupuncture points

Anti-allergy point
Foot
Stomach
Anti-aggression point
Tongue
Eye
Liver
Spine
Lung

The needles used are sterile and disposable and made from stainless steel. Long needles are occasionally inserted parallel to the surface of the body to stimulate many adjacent points on a meridian.

The 'plum blossom needle' is a smaller hammer with fine needle spikes at its head. It is used to stimulate large areas of the body by gently tapping acupuncture points. It is virtually painless and particularly useful in children. Many practitioners are now increasingly using 'electroacupuncture' – needles boosted by connection to a small battery. Acupuncture points can also be stimulated by weak laser beam.

Trigger or 'myofascial' points are tender areas that occur in muscle and tissue, and can sometimes be felt as small knots. Needling these trigger points directly is often used in pain relief. The effects of acupuncture can also be increased by warming the needle using moxa wool placed on the top of a needle and set alight. As the wool smoulders, heat is conducted down to your acupuncture point. Sometimes the practitioner will light a 'moxa stick' and move it up and down near the skin. This practice is known as 'moxibustion'.

Cupping is another needle-free technique that many acupuncturists use. Small glass cups are warmed by burning cotton wool soaked in alcohol for a few seconds inside the cup. The cup is placed over a chosen acupuncture point. As it cools a vacuum forms inside the cup and the underlying skin is sucked up.

Once you have completed the initial 'course' of acupuncture you can be taught simple acupressure techniques until the next 'top-up'. However, there are certain points that must not be used in pregnancy. Only use the points that are taught by your practitioner or that have been mentioned in this book.

Traditional acupuncturists will also look at your tongue and feel your pulse to determine the imbalance in the flow of the internal energy or chi. A traditional diagnosis may also *sound* very different to an orthodox one. For example, back pain in pregnancy may be described as 'stagnation of chi in the channels around the back and a yin deficiency'. Thrush (candida) is considered to be a problem of 'internal damp'.

A traditional acupuncturist may also advise you on nutrition and lifestyle changes.

Q&As

Q: *Are there any problems that can occur with acupuncture?*

A: There are *very few*. Acupuncture is a very safe method of treatment as long as it is carried out by a registered practitioner. Many people worry about infections such as Aids or hepatitis being passed on. Now all acupuncturists use disposable needles that are thrown away after single use. There have been a few recorded cases of a collapsed lung (pneumothorax) after a needle was passed too deep into the chest but this is extremely rare.

After the needles have been removed the skin does sometimes bleed, but pressing on the spot with a cotton wool ball for a few seconds is all that's required to stop it. You can also feel light-headed after the first session of acupuncture. If you do suffer wait until the feeling has passed before going home, especially if you are driving.

Some people find their problem (such as migraine or back pain) actually worsens after the first session. This is called a 'healing crisis' and is a reaction of your body to the acupuncture. It is often a good sign that you will respond well to the acupuncture.

Q: *How many sessions will I need and how often should I have them?*
A: Try four sessions first and pay for them one at a time. If there is no relief, stop and try something else. Depending on your problem you can have a session a week or one every three to four days. If you find acupuncture works well, have a top-up session regularly throughout your pregnancy, for example, every three to four weeks to keep the problem at bay.

Early morning sickness:	Pericardium 6
Migraine:	Liver 2
Sciatica:	Bladder 60
Back pain:	Bladder 23
Asthma:	Lung 7
Sinusitis:	Yintang point
Stress/tension/anxiety:	Liver 3
Lethargy or fatigue:	Three Heater 6
Labour pain:	Bladder 67
Dizziness:	Governor 26
Constipation:	Conception 6
Poor milk supply:	Small intestine 1

Q: *Are there any dos or don'ts when you are having acupuncture?*

A: Yes. Avoid alcohol, large meals, hot baths or showers and strenuous exercise (including sex) immediately before or after treatment, as they may counteract the effects of acupuncture.

SELF-HELP TIPS

Press on each acupressure point gently for three to five minutes.

LOCATION OF POINTS

Liver 2
On the top of the foot in the web between the big and second toes

Liver 3
As for Liver 2 but about 2cm further up toward the ankle

Pericardium 6
Middle of the wrist, two fingerbreadths below the wrist crease

Governor 26
In the middle of the furrow between the upper lip and nose

Yintang
Between the eyebrows

Bladder 67
Press the skin on your little toe (at the outer edge of the nail) with a matchstick

Bladder 60
Outside of the ankle, between the bone and Achilles' tendon

Bladder 23
Two fingerbreadths either side of the spine and three fingerbreadths above the level of the upper pelvic bone (iliac crest)

Conception 6
Three fingerbreadths below the navel in the midline

Lung 7
Two fingerbreadths above the wrist crease on the thumb aspect

Three Heater 6
Four fingerbreadths above the wrist on the back of the forearm.

Small intestine 1
Press the skin on your little finger (at the outer edge of the nail) with a matchstick

9

ALEXANDER TECHNIQUE

Frederick M. Alexander (born 1869), a Tasmanian actor, realised that the hoarseness he usually developed towards the end of long performances was because of the way he held himself on stage. He was squeezing his vocal cords by pulling his head back and down, shortening his spine, and tensing his arms and legs. Once he had taught himself to stop these 'habitual poses' by concentration and exercise, his voice and general health improved remarkably. The technique now has worldwide popularity, especially in the performing arts and among athletes.

Alexander teachers believe that the natural poise we have as children is displaced out of our bodies by years of poor posture and muscle tension. In time these stresses affect the way our muscles, joints and ligaments work, and eventually damage the whole body. Learning to stop these 'bad habits' by relearning the basics such as sitting, standing and lifting will ease the stresses on the body so that it can perform more efficiently. As Alexander said: 'If we will stop the wrong thing, the right thing does itself.'

WHAT CAN YOU EXPECT?

Early lessons are usually given on a one-to-one basis. Wear loose and comfortable clothing so that you can move easily and keep warm. The teacher will begin by showing you how to sit or lie correctly, making minor adjustments to your posture so that you know what that particular posture feels like. Further lessons involve re-educating your body to move correctly and without unnecessarily straining other muscles and ligaments. The teacher will make gentle adjustments to your posture and movements until the new movements become automatic. For example, when teaching you how to stand up correctly, the teacher may hold your head and back between the shoulder blades and you will try to stand and sit using the correct technique – using the legs for power and *not* leading with the head.

Q&As

Q: *Is there any downside to the Alexander technique?*

A: The only 'problem' with the technique is that it can take two or three months to learn the basics. Teachers also recommend that you attend a refresher course regularly.

Q: *I have heard that the Feldenkrais technique is similar to the Alexander technique. Can you tell me more about it?*

A: The Feldenkrais technique is a combination of Alexander technique, yoga, stretching and Eastern martial arts. Practitioners believe that they can change not only body attitudes but also mental attitudes – 'body psychotherapy' is a name sometimes given to this technique. Although one-to-one teaching is given, there is more group work than with the Alexander technique and pupils follow the teacher's lead of simple, basic, natural movement.

10

APPLIED KINESIOLOGY

Kinesiology means 'the study of movement'. Applied kinesiology or AK was first devised by an American chiropractor, Dr George J. Goodheart, in 1964. He discovered that testing muscle strength and tone could reveal information about patients' health and the state of their internal organs.

The system is a combination of chiropractic and the meridian theory of acupuncture: certain muscle groups are related to internal organs by the meridians that pass over them, for example the muscles surrounding the shoulder are linked to the liver, while the hamstrings are similarly 'connected' to the large intestine. Once a diagnosis has been made, treatment is given by manipulation and massage. AK is also used in the detection of allergies, and vitamin and mineral deficiencies, but this is a fairly controversial form of this practice. However, AK is becoming increasingly popular worldwide among osteopaths and chiropractors, especially those involved in sports medicine.

Touch for Health is a simplified form of AK for use by individuals in their own home and uses techniques including acupressure, massage and gentle touch.

WHEN SHOULD YOU TRY APPLIED KINESIOLOGY?

You will find applied kinesiology (AK) particularly useful for the following conditions:

- backache
- neck pain
- generalised stiffness and aches
- tiredness and malaise
- postnatal depression.

The *Touch for Health* book by John Thie (see Recommended Reading), a self-help version of AK, is also excellent for helping aches and pain, and for relaxation during your pregnancy and after your baby is born.

WHAT CAN YOU EXPECT?

There are over 40 specific muscle tests that can be carried out during an examination. Typically the practitioner will ask you to extend an arm and then will try to push down using light pressure for a few seconds. If the arm 'locks' in this position it indicates strength and health in the shoulder muscles. However, if the arm starts to shake or feels 'spongy' then a weakness may be present. More specific tests are then carried out to identify the individual muscles affected.

Once weakness has been picked up, the affected group of muscles is rebalanced by fingertip massage to restore internal energy: chi. AK is also used to detect allergies and nutritional needs. If an allergen is placed in the patient's mouth or held near the skin, muscular weakness may develop. Like many aspects of complementary medicine this allergy and nutritional testing function has not been proven but many people do find it useful. After testing you for any deficiencies the practitioner may give you a list of the kind of natural foods to eat more of so that your body is better balanced 'nutritionally'. AK practitioners can also advise on exercises to help you relax and stay calm during the pregnancy. Three to six sessions are usually recommended to get the full benefit.

Q&As

Q: *Are there any problems with AK?*

A: The one question mark against AK is that the claims made by certain practitioners can be overstated and many doctors do not actually believe in it. The only word of caution is to be very careful when taking advice about nutritional deficiencies. However, a good, reputable practitioner will only ever give you safe advice. Obviously if you are worried about a deficiency the practitioner may have picked up, talk to your own doctor about it.

SELF-HELP TIPS

Cross-crawling is easy to do and will help keep your body strong during the pregnancy and afterwards. Always start off slow and gradually build up your effort levels.

Cross-crawling is a bit like marching on the spot. It helps co-ordination and is particularly good for tiredness and aching limbs. Stand upright with feet apart. Lift the knees high towards the midline and then bring your foot back slowly to its original place. At the same time swing the opposite arm and bring your hand up to the opposite shoulder. So, as the right knee goes up, the left hand touches the right shoulder and so on. Do this for about five to ten minutes and repeat two to three times a day. You can also do this exercise to music.

11

AROMATHERAPY

Aromatherapy, along with herbal medicine, is perhaps one of the oldest therapies known, dating back six thousand years to Ancient Egypt, India and Persia. Aromatic essential oils were brought over to Europe by the Crusaders and by the Middle Ages they were being used as perfumes and medicines.

In the last 20 years it has become increasingly popular, especially in France, where over 1,500 trained doctors occasionally use essential oils as an alternative to antibiotics. Aromatherapy is a natural treatment that uses the natural oils of plants to improve and maintain well-being. Like other complementary techniques, therapists have a holistic approach and treat the person as a whole.

The oils are extracted from the flowers, leaves, stems and roots by pressing, heating, boiling or steaming the plant until it gives up its essential oil. Aromatherapy uses some three hundred different oils. Some can be very expensive due to the rarity of the plant or the fact that only a very small quantity of oil can be harvested from a large amount of the plant extract.

The action of aromatherapy on the

WHEN SHOULD YOU TRY AROMATHERAPY?

Aromatherapy is now so popular in pregnancy and labour that many midwives often give basic advice in antenatal classes. Some midwives also practise aromatherapy themselves and will use it to help you to make childbirth a positive experience. Aromatherapy is easy to learn – just follow the advice for the various ailments in the self-help tips section below.

The advantages of aromatherapy are that the basics are easily self-taught from books or local courses.

state of mind depends on the link between smell and memory. Both centres are found in close proximity in the brain and this may be why smells and aromas can activate powerful emotions (such as a sense of well-being, relaxation or fear) and strong memories. As well as this powerful psychological effect, aromatherapists also believe that essential oils stimulate the body into healing itself by penetration of the oils into the body.

WHAT CAN YOU EXPECT?

Aromatherapy is designed to treat you as a 'whole', so the aromatherapist will spend some time taking a full medical history, including personality and your likes and dislikes. Once a diagnosis has been made the therapist will then start to blend or mix certain oils with a base or carrier oil (usually wheatgerm, grapeseed or almond oil). Different personality types may receive a different blend for the same condition. Sometimes the therapist may invite you to choose your own preferred aromas. Different oils have varying properties, which may be calming, toning, regulating or stimulating. The skill of the aromatherapist is in the blending of the oils and knowing their properties and uses.

Next comes the massage, which is designed specifically to relieve tension and improve circulation. Practitioners believe this also allows oil molecules to pass into the bloodstream and eventually into the nervous system. After the massage you might experience some muscular aching and sleepiness. A body massage lasts about an hour and a facial will take 30 minutes. Occasionally you might be prescribed a few drops of oil to take by mouth daily – although this is practised quite safely, it is not advised in pregnancy.

Q&As

Q: *Are there any precautions that I need to take with aromatherapy oils?*

A: Yes, there are just a few. Never use neat essential oils on the skin, do not apply near the eyes and keep essential oils away from naked flames and children.

Q: *Are there any disadvantages to aromatherapy?*

A: Very few. Essential oils can be expensive, but when mixed in with the base oil they do last a long time. Occasionally some people get skin sensitivity, so it is important always to place a small drop of a mixture on to a small area of skin as a test before you begin using the oil.

Q: *I have heard that you cannot use certain oils in pregnancy. Which are the ones I can use?*

A: The essential oils *safe* to use in pregnancy are geranium, mandarin, neroli, ylang-ylang, grapefruit, orange, bergamot, lemon, petitgrain, frankincense, chamomile, lavender, cypress, ginger, black pepper, coriander, sandalwood, pine, rose otto and patchouli.

SELF-HELP TIPS

Aromatherapy oils should be kept in dark-coloured containers protected from heat and sunlight. Never use the oils 'neat', always mix with a base oil such as almond, sunflower, wheatgerm or avocado. Up to four aromatic oils can be used at once – mix equal quantities of the essential oils to a large volume of the base oil.

> IMPORTANT
>
> It is important **to avoid** the following essential oils in the first trimester: fennel, peppermint and rosemary.
>
> There are a few you **cannot use** at all when pregnant: sage, clove, cinnamon, clary sage, eucalyptus, fennel, marjoram, myrrh, pine, thyme, pennyroyal, camphor, parsley, tarragon, wintergreen, juniper, hyssop and basil.

Techniques to use at home

Ring burner

A few drops of neat essential oils are placed in a ceramic ring that sits on a light bulb. More than one oil can be used at the same time. Use your favourite aromas.

Oil burner

Often this is a ceramic burner that has a place for a small candle at the bottom. The candle heats a small tray or plate into which you place a few drops of oil.

SPECIFIC CONDITIONS

Back pain:
chamomile or lavender massage

Cramps:
lavender or lemon massage

Early morning sickness and vomiting:
ginger, chamomile, lavender or peppermint as
inhalations, room spray, massage or in burners

Episiotomy, tears or Caesarean section scars:
lavender compresses

Haemorrhoids:
lemon and chamomile compress

Headaches:
a few drops of dilute lavender or peppermint oil
rubbed on the temples; a lavender oil compress
placed over the forehead

Heartburn:
ginger, peppermint, lemongrass, lavender, mandarin or
coriander as inhalations or in a bath

Insomnia:
use a chamomile or lavender room spray, or try a few
drops of neroli on your pillow

Labour:
try an aromatherapy massage or bath using a
mixture of your favourite aromas

Low moods:
lavender or geranium massage, room spray or
inhalations

Mastitis:
lavender or geranium compresses

Stress and anxiety:
chamomile, lavender, sandalwood or neroli

Stretch marks:
massage twice daily can help cut these down – use
patchouli, frankincense, lavender and mandarin, either
separate or in combination. Start massaging when
you are four months pregnant (i.e. when your bump
starts showing).

Tiredness:
frankincense, ginger, lavender and patchouli massages,
room sprays or inhalations.

Room spray

Use 10–15 drops of essential oil in 100ml of water in a small sprayer. Shake well
before each use.

Baths

Add ten drops of oil to the bath water and soak yourself.

Inhalation

Add ten drops of oil to a bowl of hot water and inhale, or add a few drops to a handkerchief and inhale.

Perfume

Use diluted oil like any other perfume, behind your ears and on your wrists.

Pot pourri

Add a few drops of the pure essential oil to the pot pourri mix. Top up regularly.

Compresses

Add ten drops of oil to 100ml of hot water. Use this with a sterile gauze to the affected area three to four times daily.

Massage

Add the essential oil to your choice of base oil. You can make different concentrations, but the most commonly used is 10–15 drops of essential oils to 100ml of base oil. If you need to make a smaller quantity add 1–2 drops to 5ml of base oil.

12

AUTOGENIC THERAPY

Sometimes referred to as Western Yoga, autogenics is a method of learning to control voluntary muscles and the body's processes using deep relaxation exercises. The basic concepts of autogenics were first developed by Dr Johannes Schultz in the late 1920s. He noticed that patients under hypnosis experienced heaviness in the limbs and a general body warmth. They became relaxed and 'passively aware'. Schultz devised a system of relaxation exercises that, once taught, could enable anyone to enter this state of mind and reap the benefits of hypnosis.

Stress, the environment and disease can have an adverse effect on the body's own control processes. Autogenic training helps realign these natural processes and boost immune system function by its effects on brain-wave patterns (causing calm, relaxed, dreamy

WHEN SHOULD YOU TRY AUTOGENICS?

The secret of autogenics is that the more you practise the better you become and the more 'automatic' it is. The best time to start learning the technique is as soon as you know you are pregnant or even when you are thinking about starting a family. Autogenics is particularly good for:

- early morning sickness and vomiting
- stress and anxiety
- high blood pressure (*together* with any medication your doctor may prescribe)
- tiredness
- heartburn
- low mood
- back pain
- preparation for labour – helps reduce labour pain and anxiety.

The advantages of autogenic therapy are its strong, preventive role – for some a part of daily living and, once taught, you are able to do it without a teacher.

states), the autonomic nervous system (lowering pulse and blood pressure) and higher centres in the brain.

WHAT CAN YOU EXPECT?

After giving a brief medical history you may be asked to fill in a health question-naire. The teacher then carries out a physical and psychological assessment, and will want to know how motivated you are and why you want to learn autogenics. At the first few sessions you will be seen in a group of up to eight people and given simple exercises such as 'reclining' and 'simple sitting'. Together with correct breath-ing and relaxation techniques you will gradually become more 'passively aware' of your body.

With more sessions six standard exercises are taught, with emphasis on casual relaxation and passivity. These allow more control over your body's processes (see the Self-help tips below).

Practice is the key to autogenics and so at every session you will review the previous week's 'homework'. Your teacher will not concentrate on your symptoms – it is assumed that fitness and health will return as your skill in autogenics improves.

Advanced autogenics is usually taught to experienced trainees and involves more specific exercises, such as how to 'cool the sinuses'. Autogenic meditation is a type of autogenics that is particularly good for personal development and ailments such as insomnia and anxiety.

SELF-HELP TIPS

Try the following standard exercises. Start off by doing each one for no more than 30 seconds and then gradually build up the time for each one to 10–15 minutes. At the end of the session take a deep breath, open your eyes and slowly get up.

Exercise 1: Think – 'my right arm is heavy', then extend the heaviness to other parts of the body.

Exercise 2: Think – 'my hand is warm', then extend the warmth to the other extremities.

Exercise 3: Think – 'my heartbeat is slow and regular'.

Exercise 4: Think – 'my breathing is deep and regular'.

Exercise 5: Think – 'my stomach is warm'.

Exercise 6: Think – 'my forehead is cool'.

13

AYURVEDA

Ayurveda, the Indian philosophy of medicine, dates back to over 2000 BC. Ancient Hindu writings or 'Vedas' indicate that practitioners had great insight into human function and the treatment of ailments. They used basic diagnostic tools, carried out suturing after surgery, conceived the idea of bacteria and had access to thousands of herbal remedies.

Ayurveda is becoming more popular in the West and many believe that its greatest strength lies in its emphasis on the maintenance of good health and prevention of problems or illnesses before they arise.

WHEN SHOULD YOU TRY AYURVEDA?

Ayurveda works best when it is used to maintain good health and prevent problems starting in the first place. So as soon as you are pregnant see your practitioner who can give you advice and remedies to prevent morning sickness, constipation, anaemia, insomnia, indigestion, cystitis and vaginal infections. The practitioner can apply gentle massage to alleviate back problems, stress and anxiety. Of course an Ayurvedic will be able to help with ongoing problems as well. (See also Chapter 16 Herbal medicine.)

The advantages of Ayurveda are that it is safe if given by a reputable practitioner and has very few side-effects.

Ayurvedics believe that ill health is caused by an imbalance between the body's natural energies or 'doshas'. There are three types: Vata, which controls the muscle, bone and nervous systems; Pitta, which controls biochemistry and digestion; and Kapha, which controls cell and tissue growth. The practitioner aims to rebalance this energy disturbance. Furthermore, as in herbalism, Ayurvedic medicines may supply the body with vital nutrients and help get rid of toxins by stimulating the organs of excretion, i.e. liver, kidneys, bowels, sweat glands and lungs.

WHAT CAN YOU EXPECT?

As well as taking a full medical history the practitioner will also enquire about your family history, smoking, alcohol, occupation, sleep patterns, diet and your personality. Ayurvedics often carry out a very detailed physical examination and this will include looking at your eyes, your voice, urine and even your sweat. To make an even more in-depth examination practitioners also use astrology, palmistry, pulse and tongue diagnosis. Like practitioners of homoeopathy and herbal medicine, the practitioner will prescribe you a remedy to suit you as an individual. Along with the remedy (which is usually in powder form), you may also be recommended dietary advice, yoga, breathing exercises, massage, sweat baths, purgatives, enemas and even nasal cleaning.

Some practitioners use Chavutti Thirumal – a special form of Indian massage using the feet to rub down the body.

Q&As

Q: *Are there any problems with Ayurveda?*

A: Some traditional Ayurvedic medicines may still contain mercury and lead – these are dangerous and must be avoided, especially when you are pregnant. The best rule is always to go to a reputable practitioner and say that you are pregnant or might be pregnant. You may also find it difficult to find a practitioner. Although Ayurveda is becoming more popular it is still mainly practised in areas of immigrant population in the UK, such as Bradford, Slough, Southall and Leicester. It is also available in Australia, New Zealand and America where the interest in Ayurveda continues to grow. Most practitioners are called 'hakims' or 'vaids'.

14

BACH FLOWER REMEDIES

In 1930 the British physician and homoeopath, Dr Edward Bach, concluded that negative emotions such as despair, oversensitivity and fearfulness could lead to physical illness. He started to examine the effect of plant essences on different moods and emotions, and became convinced that they could be used to restore health and well-being. Eventually he was able to prepare 38 flower remedies – each one helping to counter a particular state of mind and the sorts of emotions that people face every day.

The flower remedies are prepared in two different ways. The 'sun' method involves steeping petals in water and exposing to sunlight for three hours. The 'heat' method involves boiling the flowers for 30 minutes. In each case brandy is added to the filtered water to make a mother tincture, which is then heavily diluted in a grape alcohol solution to form the Bach Flower Remedy.

Rescue Remedy is the most famous of these. It is a combination of five other remedies (cherry plum, impatiens, rock rose, clematis and Star of Bethlehem), and is recommended for stress, emotional or physical trauma and minor bruising. Practitioners believe that water becomes 'imprinted' with the healing properties of the flower on exposure to sunlight or boiling.

WHAT CAN YOU EXPECT?

Bach developed his remedies primarily for self-help use, although many complementary practitioners combine them with their own therapies. The remedies are available over the counter in most countries (except Germany where they are prescription medicines) in a 10ml or 20ml bottle with a dropper. Self-help books can be used as a simple guide for use in the home.

Q&As

Q: *Are the Bach Flower remedies suitable for anybody?*

A: The are very safe but not suitable for teetotallers as they contain alcohol. For children the remedy can be diluted in fruit juice or mineral water – four drops in half a glass.

SELF-HELP TIPS

There are several ways in which you can use the remedies. Put two or three drops on the tongue every three to four hours, or add two or three drops to water or juice and sip slowly. You can rub on lips, wrist, temples or behind ears, or add a few drops to water and use as a compress. Rescue Remedy is also available as a cream for bruising.

The following remedies are suitable for symptoms in pregnancy:

Rescue Remedy:
stress, physical, mental or emotional, fainting, trauma (take a few drops on the tongue every hour during labour); use as a compress in minor injuries or after an operation (e.g. Caesarean section, tears or episiotomy)

Rescue Remedy Cream:
bruising (after labour or Caesarean section)

Olive:
lethargy, feeling run down

Crab apple:
morning sickness and vomiting

Aspen:
apprehension, anxiety

Rock rose:
panic

Mimulus, Walnut or Star of Bethlehem:
fear

Mustard:
depression

15

CHIROPRACTIC

It was the Canadian osteopath and healer, Daniel Palmer, who laid down the principals of chiropractic in 1895. He claimed that he used it to cure a patient's deafness by manipulating some vertebrae in his neck. Palmer believed that even slight problems with the spinal column could interfere with nerve impulses and cause problems such as back pain and general muscular problems. In the last ten years chiropractic has become a very popular form of complementary therapy in the West – especially in the US.

Chiropractors believe that the spinal column is the key to the body's health and that it plays a vital part in protecting the nervous system. Misalignments of the spine caused by pregnancy, childbirth or poor posture can press on nerves and in turn cause back pain and eventually affect the entire body. Joint manipulation not only eases pain, but also helps the internal organs, glands and circulation.

WHEN SHOULD YOU TRY CHIROPRACTIC?

See osteopathy, page 154. Chiropractic in pregnancy should be carried out with great care and attention to the pregnancy. Vigorous manipulation to the back is not recommended. Always tell your practitioner if you are or might be pregnant.

WHAT CAN YOU EXPECT?

Chiropractors begin with a full medical history of your problem including trauma, injuries and past treatments. The examination is virtually identical to that in osteopathy. Your posture and spinal column will be examined at rest and on movement ('motion palpation'). The practitioner will also look for excessive mobility or, more usually, restriction in your movements. Straight leg raising, muscle assessment, leg measurement and routine neurological tests may also be carried out. The chiropractor may also take X-rays of your back to see if there is anything obvious out of place. It is best to avoid X-rays during your pregnancy unless absolutely necessary.

Chiropractors also use many of the specialist techniques that are described in the osteopathy section (page 154).

McTimoney chiropractic came about as a result of a split in the chiropractic movement. Practitioners of this therapy consider it a more faithful version of original chiropractic. The essential difference is that the McTimoney technique uses a more gentle approach, including light hand movements and the fingertips to manipulate joints. So if you find standard osteopathy or chiropractic too vigorous you might like to try McTimoney.

Q&As

Q: *Are there any problems with chiropractic?*

A: Like osteopathy, chiropractic is safe in pregnancy as long as the practitioner is not too vigorous. Occasionally the pain can become worse for a few days before easing up again.

16

HERBAL MEDICINE

The use of medicinal herbs goes back to the earliest civilisations of India, China, Egypt and Persia around 2500 BC. Many of these teachings were then taken up by Greek, Roman and Islamic 'healers'. Eventually, in the 16th and 17th centuries the art of herbalism spread to the rest of Europe from Turkey and Spain. From there it was a natural progression to North America a hundred years later.

Modern-day herbalism is probably the most commonly practised form of medicine worldwide, from villages in Asia and Africa to Native American Indians and tribal peoples in South America. An increasing number of medical practitioners in the West are now discovering the benefits of herbalism and practise it together with conventional modern medicine.

Pharmaceutical companies have always been interested in naturally occurring herbal medicines from which they can extract the main active ingredient and turn that into a drug that doctors can easily use. Herbal pharmacists have a different point of view. They argue that the complex mix of

WHEN SHOULD YOU TRY HERBALISM?

Herbal medicines can help many of the symptoms you might encounter during your pregnancy. As well as the problems listed in the Self-help tips on page 135, herbalism can also help abdominal pain (colic) and excessive wind, high blood pressure (in addition to any medicines your doctor might prescribe) and fluid retention.

The advantages of herbalism are that it is safe if prescribed by a professional herbalist (even in pregnancy and for children) and there are few side-effects.

substances present in their herbal remedies are naturally well balanced, and this makes them safe and effective.

Traditional Chinese herbalism differs from 'Western herbal medicine' mainly in its philosophy – the main idea being the rebalancing of Yin and Yang and internal energy (chi). Thus herbs are classified according to their effects on this energy flow, i.e. do they cool, heat, dry or moisten chi? Although more mineral and animal products are used by Chinese herbalists many of the herbal remedies used are the same as in Western herbalism.

Herbalists believe that their remedies strengthen the 'vital force' present in all living creatures to help maintain health and promote self-healing. Furthermore, the herbs act as a food to supply the body with vital nutrients and chemicals needed for normal function and tissue healing. Detoxification also plays an important part in the cure, as many herbs speed up the action of the organs of excretion, i.e. the liver, kidneys, bowels, sweat glands and lungs.

WHAT CAN YOU EXPECT?

Before treatment begins a very detailed history is taken about your emotional function, family history, occupation, exercise and eating habits. A physical examination may also be carried out, including blood pressure, microscopic analysis of your urine and pulse and tongue diagnosis. Some practitioners use other diagnostic methods such as iridology (see Chapter 28 Other therapies).

You will be prescribed a remedy for your main ailment and this could contain up to 12 herbs. The remedy is taken in the form of a pill, powder or tincture (herb extract in alcohol/water). Occasionally the herbs are put into a teabag and the 'tea' is made in the usual way. 'Over the counter' treatments are rare and the herbalist will usually make up the remedy. Creams, lotions, oils and ointments are also sometimes used.

At the end of the consultation you will be given some dietary advice and asked to follow a simple, non-refined diet with plenty of fresh fruit and vegetables.

CAUTION:
HERBS TO AVOID IN PREGNANCY

Alder buckthorn	Dang gui	Motherwort	Senna
Angelica	Devil's claw	Mugwort	Shepherd's purse
Arbor vitae	Fern	Myrrh	Southernwood
Autumn crocus	Feverfew	Nutmeg*	Sweet flag
Barberry	Goldenseal*	Pennyroyal*	Tansy
Basil oil	Greater celandine	Peruvian bark	Thyme
Black cohosh	Juniper	Pokeroot	Tree of life
Blood root	Lady's mantle	Rhubarb	Vervain
Blue cohosh	Life root	Rosemary	Wormwood
Broom	Lovage	Rue	Yellow dock
Cascara	Marjoram	Sage	
Cotton root	Mistletoe	Sassafras	

*Except in childbirth when they are safe to use

Q&As

Q: *Has there been much research done into herbal medicine?*

A: Despite its history and popularity comparatively little research work has been carried out. There are over half a million plants on earth, but only 5 per cent have been through the hands of researchers. Fortunately, with interest increasing among the general population, research also appears to be attracting more attention.

Q: *Is herbal medicine safe in pregnancy?*

A: Herbal medicines can be very potent and should only be prescribed by a professional. If you are on long-term medication ask your doctor for advice before starting any herbal remedies. There are some herbs that you can buy and use yourself. These are mentioned in the Self-help tips opposite. You need to be extra careful with Chinese herbs as some of them contain steroids and some can even cause jaundice. Always mention to the herbalist that you are or might be pregnant.

SELF-HELP TIPS

Up to four herbs can be mixed together, using equal quantities to prepare the remedy. You can make teas or infusions of leaves and flowers with one teaspoon per cup of boiling water. Cover and leave to infuse for five to ten minutes. For roots or bark, boil one teaspoon per cup in water for 10–15 minutes. Strain the tea, adding honey if desired. Never add milk or sugar. Sip slowly throughout the day. For herbal baths, prepare the herbs as for tea. Add the liquid to bath water and soak.

The following conditions can be helped by these herbs:

Early morning sickness and vomiting:
Ginger, taken as a tea, ginger beer, crystallised or in gingernut biscuits works very well. Take some before you get out of bed first thing in the morning. Chamomile teas also work well.

Anaemia:
Add parsley to meals. Drink nettle tea.

Insomnia:
Elderflower or valerian tea. Alternatively, try soaking in a Californian poppy or passion-flower bath before going to bed.

Back pain:
Meadowsweet tea twice daily.

Stress and anxiety:
Lime flower teas three times daily.

Indigestion:
Peppermint, fennel or chamomile tea (drink no more than three cups of fennel tea daily).

Labour pains:
Raspberry tea – drink daily two months before your baby is due. This remedy helps soften the tissues along the birth canal and strengthen the contractions of the uterus. Coriander also works well – try eating three or four sprigs in a raw salad or making a tea with the seeds – start a few weeks before baby is due or at the first signs of labour.

Constipation and haemorrhoids:
Psyllium as seeds or husks – one or two teaspoons twice daily in a large glass of water or squash. Stir and drink quickly. If you leave it longer than a minute the psyllium swells up and takes on the consistency of rice pudding! It helps soften your motions and eases the pain of haemorrhoids.

Poor milk supply:
Teas from dill, fennel, cumin, marshmallow or lettuce (no more than three cups of fennel tea daily).

Postnatal wound healing, e.g. Caesarean section, tears, episiotomy:
Bathe the wound with a solution of calendula mother tincture in a glass of water.

Cystitis:
Yarrow tea or cranberry juice.

Vaginal infection:
Calendula/marigold soaks.

17

HOMOEOPATHY

Homoeopathy has become one of the most popular complementary medicines to be used in pregnancy because it is very safe and also because it has so many applications.

The main ideas of homoeopathy were put forward by Dr Samuel Hahnemann, a prominent German doctor in the late 18th century. Using himself as a guinea-pig he discovered that cinchona bark, the standard treatment for malaria at the time, actually gave symptoms of malaria to a healthy person if taken in high enough doses. Hahnemann concluded that it was cinchona bark's ability to cause a malaria-like illness that made it effective against the illness. This process of 'like cures like' was explained by Hahnemann in terms of the presence of energy in every substance helping to revitalise the energy in the sick individual and so helping to cure them.

Homoeopathic remedies are made safe by diluting substances down thousands, sometimes millions, of times. Homoeopaths believe that the more they dilute down a substance the stronger or more potent it becomes ('less is more'). This is not as odd as it first appears – take the example of

WHEN SHOULD YOU TRY HOMOEOPATHY?

Homoeopathy is very safe and can help a lot of the symptoms you might experience during pregnancy, in labour and during your postnatal period. If you are a vegetarian, note that some remedies are animal based, Sepia (cuttlefish ink), Lachesis (snake venom) and Apis Mellifica (bees). See Part One of this book and the Self-help tips below to see which specific ailments homoeopathy can help.

The advantage of homoeopathy is that there are very few side-effects. Occasionally, homoeopathy produces skin changes (such as rashes or boils) or diarrhoea and catarrh. This often indicates that the body is starting to heal itself.

modern-day vaccines which are viruses so highly diluted that they do not cause disease but do stimulate the body's defences. Some remedies are so dilute that most of the molecules have been washed away. However, homoeopaths believe they still work because there is an 'imprint' of the original substance left in the remedy. Some homoeopaths have put forward the theory that perhaps homoeopathic substances are involved not in chemical reactions but merely in the transfer of information by a few molecules. Others believe that remedies may act by normalising energy flow in the body.

WHAT CAN YOU EXPECT?

After a detailed history of your problems the homoeopath will go on to analyse your general health and constitution. Patients with the same problem but different personalities and habits may well require different remedies. The range of questions asked include: family and social history, preference of temperatures, types of food preferred, personality, sleep patterns and allergies. When the therapist has built up a detailed picture of you a remedy can be chosen. These are often available over the counter from chemists or a homoeopathic pharmacist. Many homoeopaths will prepare the remedy at their practice. A calculated number of drops of the remedy are added to a quantity of sugar pills that are then taken as directed. Occasionally you may just be given drops to take. The dilution (or potency) of the remedies is varied according to the problem that is being treated. If you buy the remedies from a pharmacist they will be labelled with numbers and letters that tell you their potency, e.g. 6c, 30c and so on. 6c means that there is one measure of homoeopathic substance to a million measures of alcohol – that's like *one* grain of salt in a large bath of water, while 30c is a greater dilution still! C is the potency that is best for self-administration, but when you buy the remedy or read about it in books the 'c' is often omitted so that it might appear as Ipecac. 6 for example.

You must be careful with the homoeopathic remedies and take them in a specific way. For pills, avoid exposure to sunlight or strong smells. Avoid touching the pills as sweat makes them ineffective. The pills should be *sucked* not swallowed – the effects of homoeopathic remedies are thought to be increased by absorption through the lining of the mouth. Do not take anything by mouth 20 minutes before or after a pill (even toothpaste or drinks). The pills can be destroyed by X-rays (avoid passing them through airport security machines). For drops or liquids, hold in the mouth for ten seconds before swallowing.

You will usually be given one remedy at a time. The homoeopath will see you again after a course of pills. If you are no better you may be questioned again and try a different potency or remedy.

Side-effects with homoeopathic remedies are very rare. Occasionally your symptoms may worsen. This is thought to be a good sign but often means that the body is being over-stimulated. You should stop taking the pills for one week or until the symptoms settle, then start again.

Children often like taking tablets, but if not you can buy homoeopathic remedies in a liquid version also. Three drops are the equivalent of one tablet.

Q&As

Q: *Has there been much research into homoeopathy?*

A: Homoeopathy is one of the few complementary therapies that has had some serious research carried out on it by Western doctors. Many of the studies were done on hayfever and allergies, and show that homoeopathy does actually work.

Q: *Is there any time when you should not take homoeopathic remedies?*

A: Not really. Homoeopathy is so safe that it can be taken by anyone at virtually any time – it does not interfere with other medication. Some practitioners recommend that you take a homoeopathic remedy if you bled during the pregnancy, but the first thing to do if you do bleed is to contact your doctor straight away, especially if you have abdominal pains also. You might need a scan that day or even hospital admission, so do not delay.

Q: *Is homoeopathy expensive?*

A: It can be and this is usually because the practitioner has to spend a long time at the first consultation taking a very detailed history from you. The remedies you are given can add quite a bit to the price. Some people just need the one session, while others might need up to six. The Royal Homoeopathic Hospital does see NHS patients who have their treatment paid for by fund holding practices – however, most patients (99 per cent) will have to pay for their homoeopathy privately. Fortunately, remedies are also available from local chemists, homoeopathic pharmacists and healthfood shops. It is worth using the self-help ideas in this book to see if they help.

SELF-HELP TIPS

During pregnancy take the tablets twice daily for up to ten days. This can be repeated every month though if required. If the first remedy does not work, try the others suggested.

Early morning sickness and vomiting:
Ipecac. 6c, Nux Vomica 6c, Sepia 6c

Back pain:
Arnica 6c, Bryonia 6c

Food cravings:
Chocolate (Nux Vomica), ice cream (Phosphorus), salt (Natrum Muriaticum), fish (Lachesis), odd cravings (Lyssin), bitter (Sepia). Take a 30c tablet whenever you get a craving

Sciatica:
Ruta 6c

Feeling sore and bruised from baby's kicking:
Arnica 6c

Anaemia:
Ferrum Phosphoricum 6c or Kali Sulphuricum 6c

Heartburn and indigestion:
Carbo Vegetabilis 6c, Kali Muriaticum 6c, Pulsatilla 6c

Constipation:
Nux Vomica 6c, Natrum Muriaticum 6c

Haemorrhoids:
Arnica 6c, Arnica cream, Sulphur 6c, bathe anal area with Calendula mother tincture

Vaginal discharge:
Sepia 6c, Pulsatilla 6c

Braxton Hicks contractions:
Cimicifuga 6c

Pain relief during labour:
Arnica 30c, Aconite 6c or Chamomilla 30c

Caesarean section operation:
Arnica 30c, take immediately before the operation and another dose as soon as possible afterwards; Phosphorus 6c, helps prevent post-operative vomiting if taken before the operation

Episiotomy, tears and Caesarean scars:
Calendula mother tincture, bathe in a diluted solution, apply Calendula ointment to the scar and bruised tissues afterwards and take Arnica 6c by mouth. Alternatively Arnica cream can also be applied to the area

Low mood:
Natrum Muriaticum 6c

Cracked nipples:
bathe nipples in diluted Calendula mother tincture and apply Calendula ointment after breast feeding – wash them with water before starting the next feed or take Silica 6c by mouth

Mastitis:
Belladonna 30c, Bryonia 30c or Phytolacca 30c

Poor milk supply:
Lac. Caninum 6c, Pulsatilla 6c or Urtica Urens 6c

18
HYPNOTHERAPY

Like other complementary therapies, such as acupuncture or homoeopathy, hypnosis has a long history – the ancient Egyptians and Greeks are said to have used healing trances.

Anton Mesmer (1734–1815), an Austrian physician, was the founder of hypnosis and was probably the first medically qualified doctor to use the technique – hence the phrase 'to mesmerise'. A century later doctors suggested this therapy was called 'hypnotism' after the Greek word meaning 'sleep'. Hypnosis has recently seen an upsurge in the UK, largely due to the huge popularity of television stage hypnotists in action among a studio audience. Apart from its entertainment value, hypnosis also has a great deal to contribute to modern medicine.

Hypnotism targets the subconscious part of the mind to try and make it more receptive to suggestion. Both the patient and practitioner have to work together to make it work. The patient has to *believe* in the idea and *expect* it to work. It also helps to have a good *imagination*. The practitioner's role is to talk and *misdirect* attention – the patient concentrates her attention upon something irrelevant to the actual hypnosis such as a coin, a watch, a fantasy etc. So with her mind focused on the 'diverting channel' she is unable to harbour doubt and quickly falls into a 'trance'. Hypnosis is often described as a condition *like* sleep but not actual sleep. The patient is never unconscious. It may be better described as a condition of considerably increased suggestibility. Patients who request the therapy *allow* themselves to be hypnotised.

Hypnotism seems to work well for pain relief and helping addictions (such as smoking) by placing the uncomfortable sensations in a level of consciousness that is separate from central awareness. It is rather like driving a car: you are not aware of every sensation and action; you drive but you do not notice the driving.

WHAT CAN YOU EXPECT?

The practitioner will take a brief history of any problems you might be having. It will be emphasised that hypnosis is not a cure – rather it helps you to help yourself. Putting someone into a hypnotic trance is called induction. There are almost as many induction techniques as there are practitioners. The particular one used depends on the practitioners' experience and your personality. Some of the common methods of induction used include the following.

Arm levitation

The practitioner induces your arm to move and the hand to caress your face. Your arm then drops down to your lap and you find yourself sinking further into a relaxed state.

Eye fixation

You are asked to fix your gaze at an object (e.g. a watch, circle or point on the ceiling) while the practitioner speaks.

Visual imagery

You imagine a blackboard with a box of chalk and a duster. You are asked to draw something simple on the board and then rub it out. Many patients actually draw in thin air during this technique – a good sign of a deep trance.

The dropped coin technique

You hold a coin to concentrate and feel while you are talked through the hypnotic state. When the coin drops your eyes will close and the body will become relaxed.

Relaxation through release of tension

The practitioner asks you to tense different parts of the body while being induced. You may be asked to press firmly on the ground or hold an arm rigid. You are then asked to quickly release the tension – you should feel relaxed, rather like a stretched-out rubber band relaxes when let go.

Eye closure

You close your eyes and relax deeply while the practitioner tries to induce a trance by talking to you. During your induction you will usually move through different stages of hypnosis, namely light, medium and deep trance. The practitioner may also deepen your trance by asking you to count numbers or by breathing deeply.

A typical induction may sound like this:

> *You are comfortable and relaxed in your chair. As you sit with your hands lying easily in your lap start counting out slowly from five to one. With each number you will feel yourself relaxing more and more. Gradually the numbers will become fainter and fainter so that by the time you reach one you will barely be able to say the number. Your eyes will close and your whole body will sink down deeply into the chair. You will feel completely at rest and absolutely relaxed.*

The hypnotist will speak to you in a slow, monotonous tone while repeating key sentences to reinforce the suggestion. During the trance you might be asked to give a further, more detailed history to gain a deeper insight into your problem.

After a session you may 'suffer' from amnesia or any one of the numerous suggestions that the hypnotist has implanted in your subconscious such as hallucinations or sensory phenomena (e.g. an itchy nose). This post-hypnotic suggestion is one of the most useful techniques in hypnotism. Your practitioner may also teach you self-hypnosis and this is very useful in relieving pain and boosting confidence.

Q&As

Q: *I am afraid that while I am under the trance I could do something that I don't want to. Is this common?*

A: Many people are worried about this, but it simply does not happen. You are fully in control and can hear everything that is being said. You can accept or reject anything that is suggested. Your conscience will not allow you to do anything that goes against your own moral and ethical principles.

Q: *Can anyone have hypnosis?*

A: Almost anybody, but you should avoid it if you suffer from severe depression, epilepsy or a psychosis such as manic depression or schizophrenia.

SELF-HELP TIPS

Autosuggestion is often very helpful and just involves repeating a simple, positive statement. Try saying 'I will be calm' or 'I feel confident' or 'I am not afraid'.

19

MASSAGE

Massage is a complementary therapy that has been used throughout the ancient cultures of India, Persia, China, Arabia, Egypt and Greece. Although there are over 80 different types of massage the most modern techniques are derived from Per Henrik Ling's (1776–1839) practice of 'Swedish' or 'classical' massage.

Massage is often used together with other therapies (e.g. osteopathy, polarity, aromatherapy, rolfing, reflexology, shiatsu and kinesiology) and is currently enjoying re-emergence as a therapy in itself.

Massage has many benefits – particularly its ability to ease muscle tension, stretch scar tissue, break down adhesions and increase blood and lymph circulation. In common with other mammals, humans find the act of touching very comforting. The psychological benefits of 'massage touch' undoubtedly contribute to its therapeutic effect and this is probably because the body releases some of its natural painkillers (endorphins).

WHEN SHOULD YOU TRY MASSAGE?

Massage is one of the best therapies to use in pregnancy because it is so safe and it is easy to learn the basic techniques. Massage is particularly good for:

- back pain, sciatica, aching joints, muscle stiffness and cramps
- psychological problems such as anxiety, stress, insomnia, depression, feeling down
- preparation for labour: your chances of having an episiotomy or tearing during labour will be reduced (see Self-help tips)
- high blood pressure, but keep taking any medication that your doctor has prescribed
- labour pain, especially back pain and helping some of the anxiety and stresses during those difficult few hours.

The advantages of massage are that people can often experience positive emotional changes, it is easy to learn the basics and very little equipment is needed.

WHAT CAN YOU EXPECT?

Ideally a massage should always be carried out on a firm couch and at a comfortable room temperature. Basic carrier oils (see over) or talcum powder are used. Practitioners employ lots of different techniques, but the most common include:

- Effleurage: slow, gliding strokes using the palms, fingertips and ball of the thumb. The knuckles or thumbs are used to give a deeper massage.

- Percussion (or Tapotement): sharp, fast, stimulating movements to tone and strengthen muscles. Movements are usually delivered with the side of the hand or fingers and include cupping and clapping.

- Friction (or Frottage): deep massage by a series of small, circular movements made by the thumbs, fingers or heel of the hand.

- Petrissage: deep, vigorous, sometimes painful massage by kneading and squeezing between finger and thumb like a baker with dough.

Q&As

Q: *Are there any times when you would not recommend massage?*

A: Yes there are: massage should be avoided in people who have a fever or an infectious illness (e.g. bad flu). Also massage should not be done over areas of varicose veins, thrombosis, phlebitis, skin rashes, boils, swellings, burns or broken bones. Massage of the abdomen should not be done for the first three months of pregnancy. Also, make sure you only use the oils recommended for pregnancy (see Chapter 11 Aromatherapy).

Q: *Does it actually work?*

A: Definitely. Lots of research has been done all over the world that shows massage benefits all kinds of people, including cancer sufferers, diabetic children, teenagers with eating disorders and premature babies. Lots of nurses, physiotherapists and midwives are learning these techniques to help their patients.

Q: *How many sessions should I have?*

A: As many as you like or can afford. Better still learn some of the techniques yourself and teach your pregnancy partner also.

SELF-HELP TIPS

You can easily massage yourself although it is not as relaxing as being massaged by someone else. Gentle massage can easily be learnt by your partner and is probably the best way of easing the pains, anxiety and stress of pregnancy and labour.

Massage oils

The oils used in massage are very easy to make at home. Simply add one or two drops of essential oil to 5ml (a teaspoon) of a base oil, e.g. sweet almond oil, wheat-germ oil or avocado oil. Always buy a good quality, *pure* essential oil. Good oils for massage include lavender, geranium, rose and jasmine. You can even use different combinations of these oils, but adding two drops of each to 5ml of the base oil. See also Chapter 11 Aromatherapy.

Perineal massage

Massaging the perineal area (the part of the body between your rectum and the vagina) every day for two months before your baby is due will help soften and stretch the area and make it less likely to tear during labour. Your chances of having an episiotomy will also be reduced. Massage will also soften old episiotomy scars.

GIVING A MASSAGE TO YOUR PARTNER

- Use a firm bed or put a large towel on the carpet. Make sure the room is warm and comfortable. Use soft music and lighting to create a more relaxed atmosphere.
- Warm the massage oil before use by putting the bottle in a bowl of warm water. Alternatively, warm the oil by rubbing a little in your hands. If you do not have oil talcum powder also works well.
- Ask your partner to lie on her back or her side or whatever position is most comfortable. In labour she can lean forward and use a bean bag or pillows to support herself.

- Cover your partner in two large towels. Uncover the area to be massaged, then re-cover before moving on to the next part of the body. This keeps your partner warm and comfortable.
- In general, begin by massaging the back, neck and back of the legs, shoulders, arms, hands, neck and finish off at the face.
- Start off gently. As a general rule always massage towards the heart using long, flowing strokes. Keep one hand on her body at all times.
- Ask your partner what she likes and what she does not. This is especially important in labour when things can change very rapidly.
- When you are about to end the massage slow down and stop over a few minutes.

- The best time for a perineal massage is after a warm bath, when the tissues are soft and more elastic.

- Use a simple base oil only, such as wheatgerm, almond or olive oil.

- Gently insert two fingers into the vagina and press towards your rectum. Massage the back wall of your vagina, following the U shape of your body. Increase the space between your fingers so that the skin slowly stretches. Concentrate also on any old episiotomy scars, massaging them gently from both the inside and outside of the vagina.

- As you get nearer the delivery date you will find that you can insert more of your fingers, and that the perineum and the surrounding skin will soften and stretch even more in preparation for the birth of your baby.

MASSAGE IN BABIES

Giving a baby a massage is as much fun for the parents as it is for the baby. Massage will also strengthen the special bond that exists between you and your baby.

- As with adults use a warm, comfortable room and a nice, soft towel. Put some soft music on in the background, or you can also hum or sing to your baby. Keep maintaining eye contact as much as possible.

- Remove anything that might scratch your baby such as a watch or jewellery.

- It is best to avoid essential oils on children younger than 12 months as their skin is very sensitive. Instead, use simple baby oil, almond oil or olive oil.

- Start with your baby lying on her back. Warm a few drops of oil in your hands and start at her chest, using gentle circular motions with your fingers or thumb. Move down to her abdomen and then on to her arms, legs and eventually her back. As you get more confident with the feel of your baby giving her a massage will become easier.

- At the end of the massage remove her excess oil with a towel and do be careful when you pick her up as her skin will be slippery.

20

MEDITATION

Meditation is a systematic method of helping induce relaxation, inner harmony and increased awareness. Meditation is practised in almost all of the world's major religions. Muslims practise a form of meditation five times a day when they face Mecca and recite prayers from the Holy Qur'an.

Followers of Buddhism incorporate forms of meditation into their daily lives. Hinduism, particularly, has contributed many forms of yoga and meditation.

However, meditation can be practised without religious or spiritual associations. In fact most people go through a form of meditation regularly – getting lost in your own thoughts, listening to a piece of music, engrossed in a book... Systematic meditation takes many forms and there are a number of different philosophies and schools of thought. However, they all have the same goal – to approach and understand higher levels of awareness, and to use the experience to gain physical and

WHEN SHOULD YOU TRY MEDITATION?

Like autogenics the best way to use meditation in pregnancy is to start early – preferably before you have even conceived. The more you practise the better you become. Meditation will keep you healthy and happy if you practise for at least 20 minutes every day (see Self-help tips below). It can be used for the same specific ailments as autogenics, namely:

- early morning sickness and vomiting
- stress and anxiety
- high blood pressure (continuing any prescribed medication)
- tiredness
- heartburn
- low mood
- back pain
- preparation for labour – helps reduce labour pain and anxiety.

The advantage of meditation is that it is easy to learn.

psychological benefits. For many meditation is not simply a therapy, it is a way of life.

The increased awareness during meditation has been shown to be associated with a definite pattern of electrical activity in the cerebral cortex or the 'thinking' part of the brain. The brainwaves associated with this electrical activity are called alpha waves. Similar waves are found in calm, relaxed, dreamy states such as sleep, but the waves during meditation are much greater in intensity. These brainwaves may in turn have a beneficial effect on the body's natural control processes, slow down the heart rate and lower blood pressure.

WHAT CAN YOU EXPECT?

Your teacher will act as a guide and take you through simple methods of meditation first, moving on to different techniques to achieve 'higher planes of awareness' or to help with any specific problems. The basic lessons involve sitting comfortably, learning to relax different muscle groups and breathing exercises. Chants or mantras (a word or phrase repeated continually) such as 'om' are occasionally used to aid meditation. The mantra occupies the mind and the vibration of sound helps concentrate energy. Other methods to help focus the mind include visual images (such as a candle flame or flower bud), aromatic oils, burning incense and listening to soothing music. Meditation has also been used to help people suffering from illnesses such as asthma, cancer, ischaemic heart disease and chronic pain. The most popular form of meditation in the world is transcendental meditation or TM. This was popularised by Maharishi Mahesh Yogi (and the Beatles!) in the US in the 1970s. TM is based on Hindu teachings, through the repetition of a mantra.

Most sessions will last 20–30 minutes and are usually done in a group. A basic course will last 7–10 sessions. You will also need to practise daily at home for at least 20 minutes. You can also learn it easily from a book, video or cassette tape.

Visualisation for relaxation

- Once you are comfortable in your chair, close your eyes.
- Allow a favourite image to develop in your mind, such as the ocean, a waterfall, the beach, a painting, etc.

- Gradually fill in the detail of the picture with colours and objects. Imagine as much detail as you can of each object.

- Use all of your five senses to 'fill in the picture': signs, sounds, smells, touch. Imagine your favourite colours, foods and people in this 'daydream'. Some people ask themselves questions: Is that the sun I can feel on my back? Can I hear the waterfall? What's that cooking on the BBQ? And so on.

- After 10–15 minutes let the image go and bring your attention back to your breathing, your body and eventually to your room.

Q&As

Q: *I have heard of another type of meditation called laughing meditation. It sounds like fun. What is it?*

A: This is a relatively new form of meditation that can be carried out alone or in groups. It consists of three 15-minute exercises – stretching, laughing and silence. Participants often describe feelings of deep relaxation and unburdening.

Q: *Is meditation suitable for everyone?*

A: Yes, almost everyone. Rarely it can cause disorientation, feelings of unreality, hallucinations and increased alienation from society and negativity. Therefore, deep meditation is not recommended to those who have severe depression or a mental illness such as manic depression or schizophrenia.

SELF-HELP TIPS

- Find a quiet place – you will need 10–20 minutes.
- Find an upright chair and sit comfortably.
- Keep your head, neck and body erect.
- Close your eyes.
- Place your hands on your knees.
- Gradually deepen your breathing.
- Breathe from your stomach.
- Concentrate on gentle inhalation followed by exhalation.
- Move your concentration to your forehead.
- Relax your forehead muscles. Gradually work your way down to eyes, jaw, tongue, shoulder, arms, hands, fingers, chest, abdomen, upper legs, knees, calves, feet and toes. Relax each in turn.
- Keep breathing smoothly and slowly.
- Do not try to banish thoughts that may come – just ignore them; a mantra will help.
- Concentrate on your breathing.
- Music will help deepen the meditation.
- A chant such as 'Om' or 'Who' (on exhalation) will also help deepen the meditation.

21
NATUROPATHY

Naturopathy has origins that date back over four thousand years when people believed in nature's 'healing powers' and the use of naturally occurring medicines in basic foods. It became very popular during the 19th century when spa towns in Europe emphasised the benefits of fresh air, water, exercise and sunlight. Over the years other treatments have become a part of naturopathy, and some of these include fasting, herbalism, massage, osteopathy and counselling.

Naturopaths consider that the key to health is an individual's resistance and ability to overcome disease *naturally*. Modern lifestyles, by exposing us to poor diets, stress, lack of exercise, pesticides and pollution, lower the immune system and this leaves us open to attack from bacteria and viruses. Naturopaths believe that symptoms of ill health such as fevers and rashes are seen as signs of the body's vitality and its way of re-establishing health –

WHEN SHOULD YOU TRY NATUROPATHY?

Naturopathy is an excellent way of preparing your body for childbirth. In fact, since the idea behind it is a healthy lifestyle, both you and your partner could attend for a consultation and get fit together. However, if you are pregnant, do not fast or eat a restricted diet without strict supervision from a qualified naturopath. Naturopathy is particularly good in pregnancy when you are suffering from:

- nausea and early morning sickness
- constipation
- digestive problems
- tiredness
- anaemia
- thrush
- stress and anxiety.

The advantage of naturopathy is that it is safe (even in pregnancy and for children).

suppressing these symptoms might actually make the problem worse. Instead, naturopaths try to improve health by natural methods and so restore the body's natural balance or 'homoeostasis'.

WHAT CAN YOU EXPECT?

A naturopath will want to build up a complete picture of you so will ask you for lots of details on your past medical history, medications, immunisations, allergies, emotional functions and family history. You will also be asked about your smoking and drinking habits, occupation, exercise and food preferences. A physical examination of your skin, nails and hair may be followed by examination of the urine and blood. Many naturopaths also use iridology (see Chapter 28 Other therapies) and muscle testing (see Chapter 10 Applied kinesiology) to help them make a diagnosis.

For treatment the practitioner will recommend several changes in lifestyle to help your body cure itself and this advice will include dietary measures (such as fasting, restrictions and supplements), hydrotherapy/spa therapy, exercises, relaxation methods and even counselling. If your body needs a boost you might also be prescribed mineral supplements, herbs or a course of spinal manipulation. If the naturopath feels that you have too many toxins in your body you may be recommended detoxification such as clay/mud packs, steam baths and mineral baths.

Q&As

Q: *What is the difference between naturopathy and nutritional therapy?*

A: Nutritional therapy is improving your health by changing your diet. So this can mean eating more organic fruit and vegetables, eating less fat and so on. Naturopathy will give you similar dietary advice but in addition you may also be recommended exercises, yoga, hydrotherapy, relaxation and even prescribed herbal medicines. So nutritional therapy is a change in your diet whereas naturopathy is a change in your whole lifestyle.

SELF-HELP TIPS

- Drink between two and six glasses of mineral water a day to eliminate waste products from your body.

- Brush your skin with a loofah for two to three minutes daily to remove dead skin and improve circulation.

- Do deep breathing exercises three times daily for about two to three minutes.

- Go Mediterranean – a diet that includes salads, lightly cooked vegetables dressed in olive oil, fresh fruit, bread, pasta, rice, and plenty of fish and white meat, is being recognised more and more as the best diet for a healthy life (and heart!).

22

OSTEOPATHY

WHEN SHOULD YOU TRY OSTEOPATHY?

Osteopathy in pregnancy should be carried out with great care and attention to the pregnancy. Vigorous manipulation to the back is not recommended. Always tell the practitioner you are (or might be) pregnant. Osteopathy is useful in the following situations:

- A wide range of muscular and joint problems in pregnancy, especially back pain, sciatica, neck pain and headaches.
- Sacro-iliac joint pain (see Chapter 8 Acupuncture and acupressure).
- Some of the conditions that cranial osteopaths have had particular success with in children under five include birth trauma, autism, spasticity, colic and hyperactivity (e.g. attention-deficit disorder).
- Although not commonly practised, some cranial osteopaths claim they can lower the risk of miscarriage by massaging the abdomen to calm down the contractions of the uterus.
- Mild postnatal depression – cranial osteopathy can relieve tension and relieve mood.

The advantages of osteopathy are occasionally immediate pain relief and it is safe – as long as manipulation is gentle.

Osteopathy was founded by Dr Andrew Still, a US Civil War doctor, in 1874. He believed that people became ill if the body's structure got out of alignment, causing a reduction in blood circulation. He was convinced that the body could be readjusted to heal itself. In 1917 these concepts were brought to the UK by Martin Littlejohn, founder of the British School of Osteopathy. He called osteopathy the 'science of adjustment'.

Osteopathy is now one of the most widely practised complementary therapies in the West (along with acupuncture and homoeopathy). In the US osteopaths have been registered as doctors since 1972. Osteopaths believe that the musculo-skeletal system – the muscles, bones, joints, ligaments and connective tissue – plays a vital part in the health of the body. Any disturbance of this system will not only cause local pain, but also interfere with internal organs and the body's other main components, such as the nervous and circulatory systems. Poor posture, injury, stress or congenital problems can all damage the musculo-skeletal system and activate disease.

WHAT CAN YOU EXPECT?

The osteopath will begin with a full medical history including trauma, injuries and past treatments. Examination of posture and palpation of the spinal column at rest and on movement is always carried out ('motion palpation'). The practitioner looks for excessive or (more usually) a lack of mobility. Straight leg raising, muscle assessment, leg measurement and routine neurological tests may also be carried out. Chiropractors tend to use X-rays for diagnosis, whereas osteopaths use X-rays more as a back-up measure to confirm findings made on palpation. Remember to avoid X-rays and other forms of radiation during your pregnancy unless absolutely necessary.

High-velocity manipulation

A vertebra that has come out of place will usually be manipulated back into position. Your body may be placed in different and sometimes awkward positions, enabling it to be used as a long lever. Skilful manipulation is quick (high-velocity) and pain-free. Often there is an accompanying 'click'. Such 'long-lever' techniques allow the vertebra to right itself and often the practitioner uses minimal force.

Direct-thrust manipulation

Direct thrusts involve placing pressure on the affected vertebra and using a push to reposition it. A loud 'clunk' may also be heard, often accompanied by instant relief.

Articulation

This involves repeated rhythmical manoeuvres that take the joints through their normal range of movement. It can be extremely effective in restoring normal joint function and alleviating pain by stretching your muscles and ligaments, and encouraging the joints to move correctly.

Joint release

The affected joint is taken to the extreme of its range of movement. A steady force is then applied to the joint causing it to 'unlock' or 'release'.

Massage

Massage is used to treat tense muscle groups or to relax tissues that may surround another problem, such as a slipped disc. Massage is also used as a preliminary technique to ready your body for manipulation.

Cranial osteopathy

This was first described by William Sutherland in 1899. He felt that gentle manual compression and tapping of the skull could improve the circulation of cerebrospinal fluid. The bones making up the skull are still soft and separate in babies and young children. Disturbances in the flow of cerebrospinal fluid (due to birth trauma, injury or tension in the body) may be eased by cranial osteopathy. Although it has few advocates at present it is gaining more acceptance, particularly in the treatment of children under five years of age. Treatment mainly involves touching and tapping, rather than obvious manipulation of the skull bones.

Prescribed exercises

At the end of the session the practitioner may demonstrate to you certain exercises to be carried out at home. These help to maintain mobility until your next treatment. You may also be given advice on posture, work positions and methods of relaxing. Some practitioners are also naturopaths and will advise on diet and general nutrition.

Q&As

Q: *Are there any problems with osteopathy?*

A: As long as the practitioner is not too vigorous, osteopathy is very safe in pregnancy. Avoid manipulation around the abdomen especially during the first 12 weeks of pregnancy. Occasionally the pain can become worse for a few days before easing up again.

23

PILATES

Born in Germany in 1880, Joseph H. Pilates worked as a nurse in England during his internment there during World War I. Feeling frustrated at the general lack of facilities for immobilised patients, he started designing exercise apparatus for them by attaching springs to hospital beds. This system formed the foundation for his style of body conditioning and specialised exercise apparatus, which he took to New York in 1926.

Although it has been well known and used by athletes and those in the performing arts for several decades, Pilates has only recently seen a surge in popularity among the general public. Joseph Pilates was so confident in his system that he is often quoted as saying: 'You will feel better in 10 sessions, look better in 20 sessions, and have a completely new body in 30 sessions.'

The Pilates system is a programme that focuses on improving flexibility and strength for the total body without building bulk. Pilates teachers claim, however, that it is not just a series of exercises, but also a sequence of con-

WHEN SHOULD YOU TRY PILATES?

Many books and videos are available on Pilates and it is also getting easier to find a qualified teacher. You can use the technique throughout your pregnancy, but it is particularly useful for:

- back pain and poor posture
- improving breathing and concentration in preparation for labour
- exercising pelvic floor muscles for suppleness in preparation for labour
- increasing the tone of stretched abdominal wall and pelvic floor muscles after pregnancy.

The advantage of Pilates is that it is a system of safe, gentle exercises, ideal for beginners.

trolled movements that engage your body and mind. Many athletes and performers use it as a form of body conditioning, injury prevention and to help speed up recovery from soft tissue injuries.

WHAT CAN YOU EXPECT?

Pilates has over 500 specific exercises using five specially designed pieces of apparatus (some with unusual names such as the Barrel, the Cadillac or the Universal Reformer), which are used to develop power and strength in muscles and develop the body uniformly. The Pilates teacher will concentrate on your specific needs by guiding you through the programme in one-to-one sessions or closely supervised small groups. Your teacher will choose a few exercises for you and show you how to do them in the correct way without putting strain on other parts of your body. Instead of using many repetitions, the Pilates method prefers you to do fewer but more precise movements, requiring more control. Many of the exercises you are given will strength the 'powerhouse' of your body – the abdominal, back and buttock muscles. This develops a strong 'central core' that acts like scaffolding for the rest of your body, allowing it to move freely.

Q&As

Q: *How many sessions will I need?*

A: You can learn the basic Pilates exercises at home from a video or book – they are easy to learn. The number of sessions required depends on your own needs, but five or six sessions is usually enough.

SELF-HELP TIPS

Basic Pilates exercises are ideal in pregnancy as they are slow and gentle. These two exercises can both be carried out up to three times daily. The first stretches and strengthens the arms and upper body.

- Sit (in an upright chair) or stand up straight with your shoulders comfortably back.

- Hold your hands out in front of you with your elbows held at right angles and pressed against your ribs. Turn your hands so they face upwards.

- While keeping your elbows pressed against your ribs slowly move your hands outwards as far as you can go. When you get to the limit stretch both arms outwards until they are straight. You will now be in a 'crucifix' position. Hold for a count of ten.

- Bring your arms back down again slowly until your elbows press against your ribs. Then bring your hands towards the front again. You are now back where you started.

- Turn your hands so that now your palms face the floor and repeat the above steps.

- Repeat the whole process ten times.

This next exercise will strengthen your back muscles and make them more supple. It is a twisting gentle exercise that can help mild to moderate back pain.

- Lie comfortably on a mat or large towel.

- Stretch both your arms out to the sides and bend your legs so that your knees are nicely flexed and your feet are about a foot from your bottom.

- Keep your knees together or, if you find it more comfortable, hold a small cushion in between them.

- Let both your knees 'flop' gently to the right. At the same time turn your head to the left, bring your right arm over and try and touch your left shoulder. Hold for a count of ten. If you cannot reach your shoulder or you find you can go further, that is fine. Do what you feel is comfortable. But do not over stretch or strain your body.

- Now go the other way. Bring your knees to the left, turn your head to the right and bring your left arm over and try and touch your shoulder.

- Repeat ten times on each side.

24

POLARITY

WHEN SHOULD YOU TRY POLARITY THERAPY?

Polarity practitioners use a whole range of therapies which are useful for many of the symptoms you might get during your pregnancy and afterwards:

- Pain relief: backache and sciatica; sacro-iliac joint pain – located at either side of the spine just above the buttocks – caused by loosening of the ligaments in preparation for childbirth; labour pain.
- Early morning sickness: you might be given a special diet or certain herbal remedies. Always check they are safe in pregnancy.
- Headaches.
- Constipation – dietary advice will help restore the action of your bowels.
- Anaemia.
- Stress/anxiety/panic attacks/feeling down.
- Insomnia and tiredness.
- High blood pressure: if this is due to anxiety or stress – a polarity practitioner might give you a massage, a special diet and teach you relaxation exercises.

The advantage of Polarity therapy is that anything prescribed will not interact with your existing medication, but always check with your doctor if you are not sure.

A system of balancing energy flow in the body, Polarity therapy was devised by an American osteopath and naturopath Dr Randolph Stone (1890–1983). To describe the flow of energy he used the ancient Eastern concepts of chakras and the five element system. Chakras are specific areas of the body where energy is more focused (see page 173). The element system is a very old belief from India, which states that an individual is made up of five centres – fire, ether, air, earth and water. Each of these centres is linked to a different organ. Every organ is linked by this element system and can be affected by positive or negative energy flow from other organs.

By picking up the quality, nature and location of energy imbalance in the chakras and elements a therapist can diagnose the nature of the patient's ailment.

Except for a central neutral energy core, all points in the body are either positive or negative. For example, the head and right hand are positive, whereas the soles of the feet and the left hand are negative. Life energy is thought to control a person's whole life, and therefore mind and body, at all levels. The practitioner uses the hands and fingers to re-establish the normal flow of this energy and restore health.

WHAT CAN YOU EXPECT?

The aim of Polarity is to identify where the energy imbalance lies that is causing the problem. The practitioner will take a very detailed medical history and will also ask about your diet and eating habits. The way you respond to questions and your body language will also help the practitioner decide how to treat you. By taking a detailed history the practitioner can also decide the parts of your element system that are affected.

You will then be asked to remove all metallic objects and any jewellery that might be interfering with your energy flow. The practitioner will often use a wooden couch for the same reason. He will then do a very detailed examination and try to narrow down where the energy flow is blocked. He will look at your breathing, your pulse, examine your skin for areas of cold or heat and check for circulation. Lastly the practitioner will 'scan' a hand over your chakras to check their energy flow. Some practitioners also use dowsing with a pendulum and aura analysis for the same purpose.

Once the energy disturbance has been identified the practitioner will work with you to restore your normal flow by manipulation (like osteopathy), massage, exercises (e.g. yoga), relaxation techniques (e.g. meditation), dietary advice and herbal or naturopathic remedies.

Q&As

Q: *When would you not advise Polarity therapy?*
A: Because Polarity can involve massage you should avoid this part of the therapy

if you have a fever or an infectious illness. Do not have massage over the abdomen in the first trimester, nor over areas of varicose veins, thrombosis, phlebitis, skin rashes, boils, swellings, burns or broken bones. Most herbal remedies are absolutely safe in pregnancy but always tell the therapist that you are or could be pregnant or check with your own doctor.

Q: *Can you find a practitioner easily?*

A: Although it is gaining popularity, an experienced Polarity practitioner can be hard to find. See Useful addresses at the end of this book. You should aim to have about six sessions.

25

REFLEXOLOGY

Reflexology (or zone therapy) aims to treat the whole body through contact with the feet. It was widely used by ancient civilisations including the Japanese, Indians, Egyptians and the Chinese five thousand years ago. Modern reflexology was developed in the US in the early 1900s and introduced to the UK in the 1960s. Its popularity has soared since then.

WHEN SHOULD YOU TRY REFLEXOLOGY?

Reflexology can be particularly useful if you suffer from:

- Problems with conception/fertility. Although not proven many women have found reflexology has helped them conceive. This may be in part due to decreased stress and anxiety levels.
- Back and neck pain and stiff/painful joints.
- Constipation: reflexology can change the way your intestines contract. Some women get a bowel movement half-an-hour after treatment.
- Early morning sickness.
- Insomnia.
- Anxiety and stress.
- Postnatal depression.
- Feeling run down or exhausted.
- Loss of libido.

- Labour pains: your midwife might be able to give reflexology while you are in labour. If not ask your partner to learn some basic techniques in preparation for the big day. Reflexology can also shorten a long labour by stimulating the release of the hormone oxytocin, which helps the uterus to contract.
- Migraine or tension headaches.
- Restless legs.
- Overdue pregnancy: some mothers have tried natural induction by reflexology to start off labour when they were more than two weeks overdue. The technique may work for some by increasing the baby's movements.

The advantages of reflexology are that it is gentle, calming and revitalising, and it is a portable skill that is easy to learn.

There are areas or reflexes in the feet that represent all parts of the body. The reflexes are found on the sole, side and top of each foot. The right and left feet represent corresponding areas of the body from the 'top down'. Thus the toes represent the brain and sinuses, the digestive tract is in the middle of the foot and the heel represents the genitalia. Similar reflexes are found in the hand, but the feet are preferred because they are more sensitive and the reflex areas are larger.

The traditionally held belief is that energy flows through the body vertically from the head to the feet in specific zones. Reflexologists believe that when there is an imbalance in the body, waste matter, in the form of uric acid crystals, builds up in certain reflex areas in the feet. These crystalline deposits feel like granules and are thought to interfere with nerve impulses. Massage clears the problem by breaking down the crystals, promoting nerve transmission and allowing the body's 'internal energy' to circulate freely.

Practitioners also believe that massage improves blood and lymph circulation to the corresponding part of the body and regular reflexology activates the body's natural healing ability.

An increasing number of nurses and midwives are now practising complementary therapies, particularly reflexology and aromatherapy.

WHAT CAN YOU EXPECT?

After taking a full history of your health and lifestyle your feet will be examined in the practitioner's lap, looking for any signs of infection, presence of hard skin, corns, verrucae, state of the nails, scars or injuries, swelling, temperature, colour and perspiration. Before the main treatment your feet are readied by a gentle massage using talcum powder.

The practitioner will use several techniques to massage your feet. The thumb is held bent and the side and end of the thumb are used to apply firm pressure on a reflex point that can be no bigger than a pinhead. Creeping movements are used to move from one reflex to the next to avoid loss of contact with the foot. Some areas may feel very tender. The sensation may vary from a sharp pain to a dull ache. Reflexologists believe that pain occurs in areas of energy blockage and build-up of crystals. Treatment relieves this blockage and eventually the pain.

The practitioner will treat both of your feet and afterwards may teach you hand reflexology techniques to practise on yourself until the next session. Most people are much better after only two or three sessions, but go on to have a 'full course' of between six to eight sessions. You can have weekly sessions or several in a week – whatever suits your individual needs.

Other, similar techniques include the metamorphic technique. This offshoot of reflexology considers the foot as representative of the nine-month gestation period inside the womb. A light, feathery touch is used to help emotional problems developed during this time. This technique is particularly useful with mentally and physically disabled children.

Also, vacuflex reflexology was introduced to the UK in the late 1980s after initial development in South Africa. It uses foot reflexes and acupuncture meridians, and is ideal for patients who cannot tolerate finger pressure in conventional reflexology. Felt boots are placed over the feet from which air is sucked out to form a vacuum.

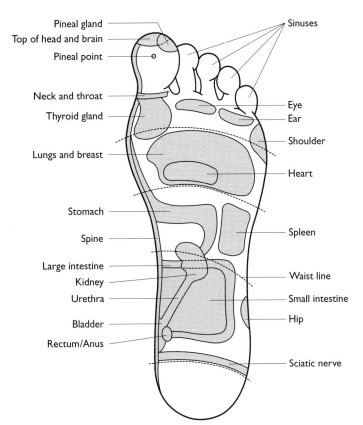

Reflexes of the sole of the left foot

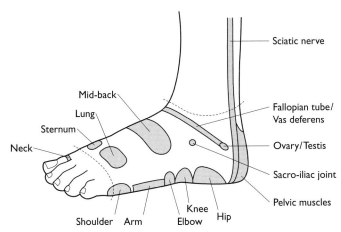

Reflexes of the top and sides of the left foot

This suction then stimulates all the reflexes. Coloured patterns remain on the feet after the boots are removed, and these last for 15 to 20 seconds. These relate to areas of congestion and infection in the body. These patterns change after each treatment and can illustrate progress made during and after treatment. The second stage of each treatment involves the stimulation of meridians running across the feet, legs, hands and arms. Silicone pads are used instead of needles and are kept in place by a gentle vacuum.

Q&As

Q: *Do some people have problems with reflexology?*

A: Most people tolerate reflexology very well unless they are very ticklish! Some patients may suffer from a 'healing crisis' after a treatment as the body fights to eliminate toxins. The symptoms are usually short-lived but can include fatigue, change in sleep pattern, increased urination, increased bowel activity, increased perspiration, increased vaginal discharge or coughing and sneezing. Fortunately this healing crisis is not very common.

SELF-HELP TIPS

For self-help, massage of the hands is often more convenient. Always massage the reflexes in both feet or hands for about ten minutes.

- To help constipation and early morning sickness use the thumb to massage across the palm of the opposite hand. Constipation can also be helped by massaging the large intestine point (see page 165).
- For help with haemorrhoids, gently massage around the inner arch of your foot where it meets the heel.
- For leg pain due to sciatica, press the reflex (found in the middle of the heel pad, see page 165) firmly with the tip of your thumb.

- For migraine, squeeze the big toe.
- For relaxation and pain relief during labour, start off by massaging the centre of your big toe (pituitary reflex), then move down the middle of your foot (adrenal reflex) and finish off at the spleen reflex (see page 165). Ask your partner to practise this technique so that he or she is ready to give it to you on the day of the birth.

26

ROLFING

Rolfing or structural integration was first developed by Dr Ida Rolf (1896–1979), who used this technique of deep massage long before the establishment of the Rolf Institute in Boulder, Colorado in 1973. Rolfers believe that stresses and strains are forced on our bodies by poor posture, injury and gravity. These distort the body's natural balance and throw it out of alignment. To overcome these structural problems, Rolfing works not by curing but by altering, correcting and re-educating the body.

The human body is an incredibly complex machine with millions of moving parts that are constantly interacting. Rolfers believe that if one part of the 'machinery' is defective it will affect the efficiency of the whole system. Deep massage and pressure is used to soften up and stretch the body's supportive wrappings (ligaments, tendons and fascia), to free them up so they can work better together. Rolfing also realigns the body and this helps gravity flow more easily. This in turn cuts down the stresses and strains caused by poor posture and injury.

WHEN SHOULD YOU TRY ROLFING?

By gently stretching and re-educating the body Rolfing can help a lot of the aches and pains many women experience during pregnancy and after the baby is born:

- back pain and sciatica
- poor posture
- stress and anxiety: Rolfing can be very relaxing particularly if you release your emotions during therapy.

The advantage of Rolfing is that patients can often experience positive emotional changes.

WHAT CAN YOU EXPECT?

The practitioners will want to know all about your past medical history, especially about any injuries or operations. You will then be assessed from all perspectives (back, front, sitting, walking, lying) to see how your body moves and works. Some Rolfers even take before and after photographs to monitor changes that take place after therapy.

By using fingers, hands, elbows and knees deep massage and pressure is given to specific areas of your body at each of the first five or six sessions. This deep massage can be uncomfortable and you might even want to let your emotions out by crying or groaning. In fact Rolfers positively encourage this! You will also be asked to assist in the therapy by breathing and moving in certain ways on the practitioner's instruction.

During the latter four or five sessions the now more flexible tissues are re-educated and each system in the body is encouraged to work with the next. You can also expect to be given specific exercises to carry out at home until the next follow-up session. A minimum of ten sessions are recommended one to three weeks apart. However, you might want to continue throughout your pregnancy and afterwards.

Another technique related to Rolfing is Hellerwork, which is a gentler form of Rolfing, with a special emphasis on the thoughts and emotions released during therapy. Aston Patterning is also similar to Rolfing, but concentrates more on movement education and gentle massage.

Q&As

Q: *Are there any times when you would not recommend Rolfing?*

A: Yes there are. If you suffer from inflammation or infection of the veins or lymphatics, or shingles, you should not have Rolfing therapy. Check with your doctor to make sure. Rolfers often do very deep massage, but always tell the practitioner that you are or may be pregnant and they will be very gentle. Rolfing is not recommended around the abdomen during the first trimester.

27

SHIATSU

Shiatsu evolved from ancient Chinese massage and is based on the concepts of internal energy (chi), Yin and Yang and acupuncture meridians. As such there is little difference between shiatsu and acupressure. Shiatsu is still commonly practised in Japan, where it is seen by many as a form of preventive health, self-treatment and boosting the body's immune system.

WHEN SHOULD YOU TRY SHIATSU?

You can easily learn simple shiatsu/acupressure techniques to help yourself throughout pregnancy. In theory, all the conditions that can be helped by acupuncture should also benefit from shiatsu. However, there are certain problems that can occur in pregnancy that respond particularly well to this technique. There are a few points that you should not use if you are pregnant – just follow the self-help guide in the Self-help tips section of Chapter 8 Acupuncture.

- early morning sickness
- migraine
- back pain and sciatica
- stress/tension/anxiety: during pregnancy it is best carried out by a professional using aromatherapy oils to relax you even further. During labour get your partner to stimulate the acupoint Liver 3 (see Chapter 8, page 113)
- Lethargy or fatigue: again best done by a professional during the pregnancy
- dizziness
- constipation
- labour pains.

The advantages of shiatsu are that it is gentle and non-invasive, and many patients feel relaxed and invigorated after treatment.

Practitioners try to rebalance chi that may be overactive, stagnant or weak, in order to let the body repair itself and stay healthy. Massage itself improves circulation of blood and lymph, breaks down adhesions and relaxes muscles. Some also claim that there is a transference of healing energy from the masseur to the patient during the process of touch.

WHAT CAN YOU EXPECT?

To try and get a better understanding of your condition the practitioner will take a full medical and personal history, and might also carry out pulse and tongue diagnosis. Then, as you lie comfortably on a mat, constant fingertip pressure is applied to various acupuncture points over your body. On larger areas pressure may be applied using hands, elbows or even feet. Occasionally some acupuncture points can also be stimulated by using certain oils during massage or by moxabustion (see Chapter 8 Acupuncture). Practitioners also claim they can regulate the flow of chi by 'opening' meridians and bringing them nearer the surface. This is achieved by placing your arms and legs in specific positions for a few minutes at a time.

There are lots of other forms of acupressure but the two you are most likely to come across are Jin Shen Do (a subtle form of shiatsu where holding or a slight pulling action is preferred) and Shen Tao, which involves lighter finger pressure over acupuncture points.

Q&As

Q: *Are there any times when you would not recommend shiatsu/acupressure techniques?*

A: Yes, there are a few. If you suffer from inflammation or infection of the veins or lymphatics, if you have a deep vein thrombosis or you have a case of shingles then you should not have any form of acupressure or massage therapy. If you are not sure check with your doctor.

For other queries see the Q&A section in Chapter 8 Acupuncture.

28

OTHER THERAPIES

We've looked at the key therapies discussed in this book, but there are many different complementary treatments available. You may find the following therapies are also of help during pregnancy and in childbirth. Some of these are less well-known, but others, such as yoga, are now commonly used in pregnancy.

BIOFEEDBACK

Biofeedback is a technique that uses information fed back from an instrument to control involuntary body responses such as blood pressure, skin temperature, pulse and blood flow. It is often used together with relaxation, but you focus on a specific response, such as lowering your blood pressure instead of relaxing the whole body. Biofeedback is being increasingly used in research and treatment by orthodox doctors, and is available already in some state hospitals. Electrodes are connected to the skin, and temperature or the amount of muscle activity around that area is shown by a series of clicks, bleeps or a pattern on a screen. You are then encouraged to use thoughts, sensations, feelings, breath control, meditation and any other means to alter the signals. By giving you this immediate feedback on the state of your body you can learn how to control certain processes. Biofeedback is particularly useful after pregnancy if you suffer from incontinence as it can help you to strengthen your sphincter muscles.

BOWEN TECHNIQUE

This is a gentle, subtle form of massage originating from Australia. It is particularly suitable for musculo-skeletal problems (e.g. back pain) during pregnancy. Therapists can also advise on home remedies for minor ailments. The practitioner uses thumbs and fingers to make rolling-type movements to the affected areas of the body to calm muscles, ease soft tissues and allow normal energy to flow in the body. During the therapy you may have periods of rest to allow your body to fully absorb the effects of the technique. Avoid Bowen massage around the abdomen in the first trimester.

COLOUR THERAPY

Visible light is made up of the seven colours of the rainbow. The eyes are sensitive to the whole range of hues, and the appreciation of colours and colour therapy was known to the ancient Greeks, Romans, Egyptians and Indians.

Today it is well recognised that colours have a strong effect on moods and emotions. Colours at the red end of the spectrum make the body tense and excitable, whereas the blue end colours are calming and relaxing. Colour also affects our perception. A blue room appears larger than a red one. Each colour has a characteristic energy level, as does every living cell. Practitioners believe that disease or illness can cause deficiency in this energy. Exposure to a colour with a similar energy pattern might redress this imbalance and help emotional and physical problems.

The therapist will ask about your favourite colours, most disliked colours and also about your particular ailment to see which colour energies are still strong. The therapists will use several techniques to diagnose which colour energies are lacking. Aura and chakra analysis are the most popular used. The human aura contains seven colours that extend out from red-orange-yellow-green-turquoise-blue-violet to magenta. Change in shape and

SELF-HELP TIPS

- Tired and lethargic: wear bright colours, e.g. orange and yellow.
- Insomnia: paint your bedroom green or put up green curtains and move in plenty of plants.
- Fed up, bored at work: put an orange object on your desk.
- Worried about someone or something: visualise them or it bathed in blue light.
- Practice visualisation meditation (see Chapter 20) and place particular emphasis on your favourite colour.

colour of a patient's aura can indicate certain problems. Chakras are areas in the body through which energies flow. They act like a lens and collect and accentuate light around the body. Each chakra is associated with a specific aura colour. Therapists also ask you to choose your three favourite colours out of eight. This is called 'colour reflection grading'. The three are placed in order of preference and the choice is analysed. For example, green (1st position) means neat and efficient with an affinity for nature, whereas red (1st position) indicates an active person who is creator and initiator. A combination of therapies might be prescribed including using coloured lights and shapes, colour visualisation, colour bath (a special bath delivering light refracted through water), massage with coloured oils, coloured crystals, and coloured clothes and foods.

In pregnancy colour therapy may help with insomnia, anxiety, stress and low moods.

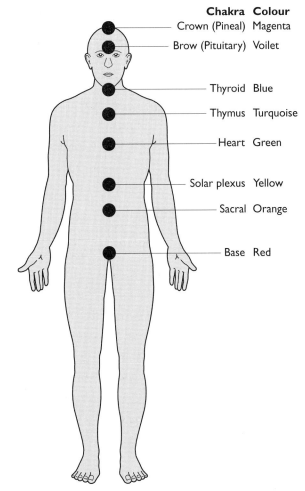

Chakra	Colour
Crown (Pineal)	Magenta
Brow (Pituitary)	Voilet
Thyroid	Blue
Thymus	Turquoise
Heart	Green
Solar plexus	Yellow
Sacral	Orange
Base	Red

Colour therapy and the chakras

CRYSTAL AND GEM HEALING

Like colours each type of crystal vibrates at a certain energy or frequency. If problems or ailments are caused by a lack of a particular kind of energy or frequency, then wearing the corresponding crystal may help to replenish and rebalance that energy. Most stones are worn close to the body, kept in the home or

SELF-HELP TIPS:
- Anxiety and stress: amethyst, blue sapphire.
- Tiredness: topaz, tiger's eye, jade, emerald.
- Back pain and inflammation: turquoise.
- Infections and general disinfectant: amber (not actually a crystal but a solidified resin).

in the car. Occasionally the stones are steeped in water and the resulting lotion used to treat disease. In ancient times crystals and gems were crushed and used as a lotion for wounds and an antidote for poison. You can pick a stone from a selection according to your ailment, personality, plans for the future and so on. Many people find that they will be attracted to a particular type of stone because of its colour and shape and choose to wear that.

FOLIC ACID

Folic acid is essential for the healthy progress of your baby in the first few months of life. It is particularly important in ensuring that the nervous system develops and grows normally. A lack of folic acid has been shown to be a cause of neural tube defects such as spina bifida ('split spine'). Sadly, almost 800 pregnancies a year are affected in England and Wales. Since 1992 the Department of Health has recommended that women planning a pregnancy should increase their folic acid intake by 400mcg a day. Women who have had an affected pregnancy can reduce the risk of recurrence by almost 70 per cent by taking 5mg of folic acid (available on prescription only); 5mg a day of folic acid is also advised in women taking epilepsy medication. The lower dose of 400mcg is recommended for women with no previous affected pregnancies. Ideally, all women should start folic acid tablets at least three months *before* conception and continue until the 12th week of pregnancy.

Some studies have also shown that folic acid may also protect against colon cancer, cervical 'pre-cancer' and heart disease.

SELF-HELP TIPS:
You can increase your dietary folic acid by eating more of the following, in addition to your folic acid tablets.

- Dietary folate: at least 50mcg per serving in asparagus, Brussels sprouts, black-eyed beans, beef/yeast extract, kale, spring greens, broccoli, green beans, spinach; 15 to 50mcg per serving in potatoes, fresh fruit, vegetables, most nuts, orange juice, baked beans, bread, eggs, milk/milk products, brown rice, wholegrain pasta, salmon/beef/game.
- Fortified foods: mainly cereals and certain breads – some of these can provide almost half your daily requirement. Check the labels.
- Avoid irradiated food: irradiation destroys folic acid.

FLOTATION THERAPY

This is basically sensory deprivation in a dark, warm, soundless tank of saline about 25cm (10in) deep and some say it is designed to mimic a person's experience in the womb. The strong concentration of salt in the water allows the body to float freely. This therapy is excellent for stress, anxiety, high blood pressure and back pain. It is not suitable for those with a nervous disposition or claustrophobia.

The therapy is available at natural health clinics and specialist flotation centres.

GARLIC THERAPY

Garlic is extensively used in the Indian subcontinent, China and South East Asia not only for its flavour but also for its health properties. It is often prescribed by complementary practitioners for the prevention and treatment of colds and influenza.

Recent research now also seems to indicate that garlic may help in maintaining healthy levels of blood fats and cholesterol. For example, taking garlic regularly may cut down clot formation, reduce blood pressure and glucose, lower blood fats and cholesterol. A substance called allicin is responsible for the taste, odour and medicinal properties of garlic. Garlic, therefore, might have a role to play in pregnancy if you suffer from high blood pressure or pre-eclampsia. As always, remember to continue with any medication that your doctor has prescribed.

> SELF-HELP TIPS:
> ● Garlic tablets are available over the counter. A special coating stops the unpleasant odour.
> ● Increase garlic in diet – raw or in cooking.
> ● To cut down the problem of garlic odour, eat with parsley, coriander, salad greens or aniseed.

Some of the side-effects of too much garlic, although rare, can be troublesome – they include a burning sensation in the mouth and stomach and occasional nausea.

HEALING

This type of therapy is also known as 'faith healing', 'spiritual healing' and 'hands-on healing'. Healers transmit energy from themselves to the patient or act as a channel for a 'universal life force'. After a gesture or ritual the healer may place a hand on or near your head. You are then asked to relax and concentrate on breathing, inner warmth and light. Sessions last for about one hour with weekly treatments. Therapists aim to rebalance energies with a *gradual* return to health.

Absent healing or healing from afar is practised if the patient cannot get to the healer due to ill health or distance. Faith is not a prerequisite for treatment and some healers have even worked successfully on animals. Most professional spiritual healers do not have religious links.

Healing is particularly good for the relief of pain and distress and is very safe. As such it is ideal for pregnancy and labour and some of the problems that may benefit include early morning sickness, high blood pressure, tiredness, low mood, stress and anxiety. Many healers do not charge for their services as they believe that it should be freely available to all.

HYDROTHERAPY

The use of water for healing and overcoming minor injuries is gaining popularity. Some of the treatments involved include jacuzzi (not recommended in pregnancy), spas, aerated pools, steam baths, sitz baths (alternate hot and cold bathing), inhalations and drinking mineral waters.

Water births have also become more popular where the mother gives birth while standing or sitting in a large birthing pool. The mother-to-be is more mobile, and the feel and warmth of the water can encourage relaxation. Many midwives and mothers have claimed that this is less painful and causes less distress to the child. There is less pressure on the abdomen, which probably allows more circulation to the uterine muscles and subsequently less pain.

SELF-HELP TIPS

Walking in a swimming pool is excellent exercise and can also help ease a bad back. Go to where the water is about chest high – walk up and down the width of the pool for 30 minutes. At the end of the session you will find that your back will ache less as the water is now supporting your weight. Aim to visit your local pool twice a week, especially in the latter half of your pregnancy. Many local pools now run aquafit classes. Start off slowly and work at your own pace. Do tell the instructor you are pregnant.

IRIDOLOGY

Iridology is a diagnostic method and involves a detailed examination of the condition, colouring and markings of the iris – the coloured part of the eye. It is believed that changes can occur in the iris long before an illness manifests itself. By detecting and analysing the causes of these early changes the therapist can recommend appropriate early treatment, together with changes in lifestyle and diet to maintain health. The technique is, however, rather controversial and as such it has no significant role in helping with problems of pregnancy. You may come across it being used as a diagnostic tool.

JIN SHIN JYUTSU

Jin Shin Jyutsu is a Japanese system of touch, gentle massage and exercises to help clear congestion in 'energy locks' and allow the free flow of internal energy or chi. As this therapy is very gentle it can help with back pain in pregnancy, as well as stress and anxiety.

KIRLIAN PHOTOGRAPHY

The basis of many complementary philosophies is that there is often a disturbance or imbalance of the body's internal energy (called chi, prana or shen – depending which philosophy you follow) that causes physical disease. Kirlian photography is a system of radiography that claims to be able to record this energy flow, which appears as an aura around the body.

A part of the body, most often the hand, is placed on to a highly charged photographic plate. Once developed the photographs show a 'halo' type effect of the hand created by the electrical interaction of the charged plate and the body's energy. It is claimed that changes in the photographs can detect changes in energy flow that *pre-empt* the onset of ill health. The technique is not without its critics, many of whom maintain that it does not have enough credibility. Kirlian photography has no real beneficial effects to contribute to pregnancy-related problems but, like iridology, some complementary practitioners do use it as a diagnostic tool.

REIKI

Like healing the basic concept of reiki is transmitting 'universal energy' from the healer to the patient. Gentle touch allows universal energy back into the patient. All the patient needs to do is be receptive to the idea and the energy will find its way to where it is most needed. Reiki, like healing, is very safe and can be used for the same ailments in pregnancy i.e. early morning sickness, high blood pressure, tiredness, low mood, stress and anxiety.

SOUND THERAPY

People have used sounds, particularly music, naturally and therapeutically through the ages. Egyptian writings over 2,500 years old refer to music and incantations as cures for infertility and rheumatic pain. In recent years there has been renewed interest in sound therapy specifically aimed at organs, and general voice therapy in the form of chants and singing. Therapists believe that each tissue vibrates at a special frequency. A person becomes unwell because these frequencies are disturbed by environmental effects, stress and disease. The tissue is 're-tuned' by applying a vibration of the same frequency to the body. The practitioner uses various ways of applying the healing vibration such as voice, special notes and tuning forks. Patients are also advised to expose themselves to music and sounds based on certain 'healing' notes. As the tissue's frequency is corrected the patient starts to feel better. Cymatics is a special type of sound therapy, where a practitioner uses a machine to pass sound waves through the body.

A version of sound therapy, music therapy, is excellent for pregnancy-related conditions especially stress, anxiety, low mood, tiredness and high blood pressure.

SELF-HELP TIPS:
- Humming or singing regularly aids stress and relaxation
- Exaggerated yawning – tiredness – releases tension in the jaw and mouth.
- Loud groaning or sighing can help with tension.
- Listen to different music and sounds, or e.g. sacred chants or Tibetan temple music.

T'AI CHI CH'UAN

T'ai Chi Ch'uan or simply T'ai Chi is a Chinese exercise that dates back over 600 years to the Taoists. The basic form has 40 movements, while the more complex form has over 100 and can take 30 minutes to complete. The movements are simple, slow and graceful, and help improve and calm the flow of the body's internal energy, chi. Practised on a daily basis, T'ai Chi is particularly useful for general exercise, relaxation, contemplation, relief of muscular aches and pains, and stress. T'ai Chi has become so popular that it is relatively easy to find courses and evening classes in your local community.

YOGA

From its Indian origins over 4,000 years ago yoga has spread throughout the world as a therapy recognised in helping stress, improving joint and muscle suppleness, and generally improving overall health. Like many gentle 'moving' therapies yoga works very well in pregnancy, especially for backache and posture. Ideally, it is best to start learning the basics before you conceive so that you can get the most benefit when you are actually pregnant. Regular yoga will also increase the suppleness in your pelvic floor muscles, which may make labour easier with less chance of tearing or having an episiotomy. Yoga can also help the pelvic floor and abdominal muscles recover much more quickly after childbirth. If you are interested in trying this popular therapy, there are several self-help books available that deal specifically with yoga for pregnancy (see page 181 for a selection of titles).

Qigong ('chee gong') is often called Chinese yoga and like many therapies originating from the East, focuses on the balance of internal energy (or chi) to help ailments and keep the body healthy. The technique involves meditation, postures and controlled breathing.

ZERO BALANCING

This is a relatively new therapy based on osteopathic techniques and Chinese theories of energy flow. Zero balancing aims to ease muscle and joint problems by manipulation, acupressure and the rebalance of internal energy flow. It seems to work particularly well for musculo-skeletal disorders and stress.

RECOMMENDED READING

General

1. Karen Evennett, *The Essential Guide to Having a Baby*, Ward Lock (1998).
2. Tanvir Jamil, *Complementary Medicine: A practical guide*, Butterworth-Heinemann (1997).
3. Stephen Fulder, *The Handbook of Complementary Medicine*, Oxford University Press (1998).
4. Hazel Courtenay, *What's the Alternative?*, Boxtree (1996).
5. Nikki Bradford and Geoffrey Chamberlain, *Pain Relief in Childbirth*, HarperCollins (1995).

Acupressure

1. Chris Jarmey and John Tindall, *Acupressure for Common Ailments*, Gaia Books (1991).
2. Michael Reed Gach, *Acupressure*, Piatkus (1992).
3. Julian Keynon, *Acupressure Techniques*, Thorsons (1987).

Alexander Technique

1. Jonathan Drake and David Garlic, *The Alexander Technique in Everyday Life*, Thorsons (1996).
2. Glynn MacDonald and Glenn MacDonald, *The Complete Illustrated Guide to the Alexander Technique*, Element (1998).

Aromatherapy

1. Chrissie Wildwood, *The Encyclopedia of Aromatherapy*, Healing Arts Press (1996).
2. Danièle Ryman, *Aromatherapy*, Piatkus (1992).
3. Maggie Tisserand, *Aromatherapy for Women*, Thorsons (1990).
4. Allison England, *Aromatherapy and Massage for Mother and Baby*, Vermillion (1999).

Ayurveda

1. Dr Vasant Lad, *The Complete Book of Ayurvedic Home Remedies*, Piatkus (1999).

Bach Flower Remedies

1. Judy Howard, *The Bach Flower Remedies: Step by Step*, C.W. Daniel Co. (1990).

Colour Therapy

1. Pauline Willis, *Colour Healing Manual*, Piatkus (2000).

Crystal Healing

1. Michael Gienger, *Crystal Power, Crystal Healing*, Ward Lock (1998).

Healing

1. Dr Rudolph Ballentine, *Radical Healing*, Rider (1999).
2. Roy Stemman, *Healers and Healing*, Piatkus (1999).
3. Jack Angelo, *Your Healing Power*, Piatkus (1998).

Herbal Medicine

1. Penelope Ody, *100 Great Natural Remedies*, Kyle Cathie Ltd (1997).
2. Jill Nice, *Herbal Remedies for Healing*, Piatkus (1998).
3. Stephen Tang and Richard Craze, *Chinese Herbal Medicine*, Piatkus (1995).
4. Carol Rogers, *The Women's Guide to Herbal Medicine*, Hamish Hamilton (1997).

Homoeopathy

1. Dr P. Webb, *The Family Encyclopedia of Homoeopathic Remedies*, Robinson (1997).

2. Drs Sheila and Robin Gibson, *Homoeopathy for Everyone*, Penguin (1991).

Massage

1. Clare Maxwell Hudson, *The Complete Book of Massage*, Dorling Kindersley (1998).
2. Lucinda Liddell et al., *The Book of Massage*, Ebury Press (1984).
3. Peter Walker, *Baby Massage*, Piatkus (1995).

Meditation

1. Eric Harrison, *Teach Yourself to Meditate*, Piatkus (1994).

Nutrition

1. Jean Carper, *The Food Pharmacy*, Simon & Schuster (1993).
2. Patrick Holford, *The Optimum Nutrition Bible*, Piatkus (1997).

Pilates

1. Lynne Robinson and Gordon Thomson, *Body Control: The Pilates Way*, Pan (1998).

Qigong

1. Michael Tse, *Qigong for Health and Vitality*, Piatkus (1995).

Reflexology

1. Mildred Carter, *Helping Yourself with Foot Reflexology*, Redward Classics (1969).
2. Laura Norman, *The Reflexology Handbook*, Piatkus (1989).

Reiki

1. Penelope Quest, *Reiki*, Piatkus (1999).
2. Mari Hall, *Reiki for Common Ailments*, Piatkus (1999).

T'ai Chi

1. Robert Parry, *The T'ai Chi Manual*, Piatkus (1997).

Touch for Health

1. John Thie, *Touch for Health: A new approach to restoring our natural energies*, D.C. DeVorss and Company, California (1973).

Yoga

1. Howard Kent, *The Complete Illustrated Guide to Yoga*, Element (1999).
2. Vimla Lalvani, *The Complete Book of Yoga*, Hamlyn (1999).
3. Francoise Barbira Freedman and Doriel Hall, *Yoga for Pregnancy*, Ward Lock (1998).
4. Janet Balaskas, Sandra Sabatini and Yehudi Gordon, *Preparing for Birth with Yoga*, Element (1993).
5. Wendy Teasdill, *Yoga for Pregnancy*, Gaia Books (2000).
6. Francoise Barbira Freedman and Doriel Hall, *Postnatal Yoga*, Lorenz Books (2000).

Zero Balancing

1. John Hamwee, *Zero Balancing*, Frances Lincoln (1999).

USEFUL ADDRESSES

You might find the following addresses useful as further sources of information or to find a suitably qualified practitioner in your area. Many of the associations ask you to send a large self-addressed envelope together with two first-class stamps.

UK

General

British Complementary Medicine Association,
9 Soar Lane, Leicester LE3 5DE
Tel: 01162 425406
(Provides lists of complementary practitioners)

Council for Complementary and Alternative Medicine,
179 Gloucester Place, London NW1 6DX
Tel: 020 7724 9103
(Provides lists of complementary practitioners)

The Institute of Complementary Medicine,
PO Box 194, London SE16 1QZ
Tel: 020 7237 5165
(Provides lists of complementary practitioners)

Royal London Homoeopathic Hospital,
Great Ormond Street, London WC1N 3HR
Tel: 020 7837 3091

Issue – National Fertility Association,
41 North Road, London N7 9DP
Tel: 020 7609 9061 (helpline)
(Help, information and support for infertile couples)

Women's Health Concern
Tel: 020 7251 6580 (helpline)
(Advice for women with gynaecological problems and other health queries)

Miscarriage Association,
Clayton Hospital, Northgate, Wakefield, West Yorks WF1 3JS
Tel: 01924 200799
(Support given by women and couples with personal experience of miscarriage)

Stillbirth and Neonatal Death Society (SANDS),
28 Portland Place, London W1N 4DE
Tel: 020 7436 5881 (helpline)

Help with Pregnancy and Childbirth

Active Birth Centre,
25 Bickerton Road, London N19 4JT
Tel: 020 7561 9006
Fax: 020 7561 9007
Email: mail@activebirthcentre.demon.co.uk
Website: www.activebirthcentre.com
(Provides information on all aspects of pregnancy, labour and parenting, including complementary therapies suitable for pregnancy. Also hires out birthing pools)

National Childbirth Trust (NCT),
Alexandra House, Oldham Terrace, London W3 6NH
Tel: 020 8992 8637 (helpline 9.30a.m.–4.30p.m.)
Fax: 020 8992 5929

Action on Pre-Eclampsia (APEC),
31–33 College Road, Harrow, Middlesex HA1 1EJ
Tel: 020 8427 4217

The Pregnancy Shop,
Manor View, Claydon, Banbury, Oxfordshire OX17 1HH
Tel: 0891 633473 (helpline) or 0870 166 8899
Email: info@pregnancy-shop.com
Website: www.pregnancy-shop.com
(Mail order service – natural products for use in pregnancy and after childbirth)

Twins and Multiple Births Association (TAMBA),
PO Box 30, Little Sutton, South Wirral L66 1TH
Tel: 01732 868000 (helpline)

After Childbirth

Parentline
Tel: 01702 558900 (helpline 9a.m.–9p.m. weekdays, 1–6p.m. Saturdays)
(Provides general counselling for parents and carers)

National Caesarean Support Network,
2 Hurst Park Drive, Huyton, Liverpool L36 1TF
Tel: 0151 480 1184

Continence Association,
307 Hatton Square, 16 Baldwins Gardens, London EC1N 7RJ
Tel: 020 7831 9831 (helpline)
(Confidential help from a specialist nurse on all problems relating to bowel and bladder control)

National Child Minding Association,
8 Mason's Hill, Bromley, Kent BR2 9EY
Tel: 020 8464 6164

NIPPERS (National Information for Prematures – Education, Resources and Support),
17-21 Emerald Street, London WC1N 3QL
Tel: 020 7831 9393

Lullababy Soothing Tapes,
Parish Lane, Kings Thorn, Hereford HR2 8AH
Tel: 01981 540288

Baby Soother Tapes,
JayGee Cassettes, 5 Woodfield, Burnham-on-Sea, Somerset TA8 1QL
Tel: 01278 789352

Advice on Breast Feeding

Association of Breastfeeding Mothers,
PO Box 207, Bridgwater TA6 7YT
Tel: 020 7813 1481 (helpline)
Email: abm@clara.net
Website: www.home.clara.net/abm

La Lêché League of Great Britain,
Box BM 3424, London WC1N 3XX
Tel: 020 7242 1278
Website: www.stargate.co.uk/lllgb/main.html

Single Parents

National Council for One Parent Families,
255 Kentish Town Road, London NW5 2LX
Tel: 020 7267 1361

Gingerbread,
16-17 Clerkenwell Close, London EC1R 0AA
Tel: 020 7336 8184 (helpline)

Acupuncture

British Medical Acupuncture Society (BMAS),
Newton House, Newton Lane, Whitely, Warrington, Cheshire WA4 4JA
Tel: 01925 730727
Email: Bmasadmin@aol.com
Website: www.medicalacupuncture.co.uk
(Register of doctors trained in acupuncture)

British Acupuncture Association and Register,
34 Alderney Street, London SW1V 4EU
Tel: 020 7834 1012
(Register of qualified practitioners, information leaflets and booklets)

The Royal London Homoeopathic Hospital NHS Trust
(see General addresses)

British Acupuncture Council,
Park House, 206-208 Latimer Road, London W10 6RE
Tel: 020 8964 0222
Email: info@acupuncture.org.uk

Alexander Technique

The Society of Teachers of Alexander Technique (STAT),
20 London House, 266 Fulham Road, London SW10 9EL
Tel: 020 7351 0828
Website: www.stat.org.uk

Aromatherapy

Aromatherapy Organisations Council (AOC),
PO Box 19834, London SE25 6WF
Tel: 020 8251 7912
Website: www.aromatherapy-uk.org

International Federation of Aromatherapists,
2-4 Chiswick High Road, London W4 1TH
Tel: 020 8742 2605

International Society of Professional Aromatherapists (ISPA),
ISPA House, 82 Ashby Road, Hinckley, Leics LE10 1SN
Tel: 01455 637987
Fax: 01455 890956
Email: lisabrown@ispa.demon.co.uk

Association of Tisserand Aromatherapists,
65 Church Street, Hove, East Sussex BN3 2BD
Tel: 01273 772479/206640

Autogenics

British Autogenic Society,
The Royal London Homoeopathic Hospital NHS Trust, Great Ormond Street, London WC1N 3HR
Tel: 020 7713 6336
Website: www.autogenic-therapy.org.uk

Ayurveda

Ayurvedic Centre of Great Britain,
50 Penywern Road, London SW5 9SX
Tel: 020 7370 2255

Ayurvedic Living,
PO Box 188, Exeter EX4 5AY

Bach Flower Remedies

The Bach Flower Centre,
Mount Vernon, Bakers Lane,
Brightwell cum Sotwell,
Wallingford, Oxfordshire
OX10 0PZ
Tel: 01491 834678
Fax: 01491 825022
Email: bach@bachcentre.com
Website: www.bachcentre.com

The Healing Herbs of Dr Bach,
PO Box 65, Hereford HR2 0UW
Tel: 01873 890218

Bowen Technique

European College of Bowen Studies,
38 Portway, Frome, Somerset
BA11 1QU
Tel/fax: 01373 461873
Email: bowen@globalnet.co.uk
Website:
www.thebowentechnique.com

Cranial osteopathy

International Cranial Association,
(formerly Cranial Osteopathic Association), 478 Baker Street,
Enfield EN1 3QS
Tel: 020 8367 5561
Fax: 020 8202 6686

Chiropractic

British Chiropractic Association (BCA),
Blagrave House, 17 Blagrave
Street, Reading, Berks RG1 1QB
Tel: 0118 950 5950
Fax: 0118 958 8946
Email: britchiro@aol.com
Website: www.chiropractic-uk.co.uk

The Scottish Chiropractic Association (SCA),
30 Roseburn Place, Edinburgh
EH12 5NX
Tel: 0131 346 7500

McTimoney Chiropractic Association,
21 High Street, Eynsham, Oxon
OX8 1HE
Tel: 01865 880974
Fax: 01865 880975
Email: admin@mctimoney-chiropractic.org
Website: www.mctimoney-chiropractic.org

Colour Therapy

Colour Therapy Association,
PO Box 16756, London
SW20 8ZW
Tel: 020 8540 3540

International Association for Colour Therapy,
PO Box 3, Darkes Lane,
Potters Bar, Herts EN6 3ET

Crystal Healing

The Affiliation of Crystal Healing Organisations,
46 Lower Green Road, Esher,
Surrey KT10 8HD
Tel: 020 8398 7252

Feldenkrais Technique

The Feldenkrais Guild UK,
PO Box 370, London N10 3XA

Flotation Therapy

Flotation Tank Association,
PO Box 11024, London SW4 7ZF
Tel: 020 7627 4962

Healing

British Alliance of Healing Associations,
23 Nutcroft Grove, Fetcham,
Leatherhead, Surrey KT22 9LD
Tel: 01372 373241

National Federation of Spiritual Healers (NFSH),
Old Manor Farm Studio, Church
Street, Sunbury on Thames,
Middlesex TW16 6RG
Tel: 01932 783164

Hellerwork

The European Hellerwork Association,
The MacIntyre Gallery, 29
Crawford Street,
London W1H 1PL
Tel: 020 7723 5676
Email: rgolten@dial.pipex.com
Website: www.golten.net

Bodyworkers,
Suite 211, Coppergate House,
16 Brune Street, London
E17 NHJ
Tel: 020 7721 7833

Herbal Medicine

National Institute of Medical Herbalists,
56 Longbrook Street, Exeter
EX4 6AH
Tel: 01392 426022

British Herbal Medicine Association,
Sun House, Church Street,
Stroud GL5 1JL
Tel: 01453 751389
Fax: 01453 751402

The General Council and Register of Consultant Herbalists,
18 Sussex Square, Brighton,
East Sussex BN2 5AA
Tel: 01243 267126

Homoeopathy

Faculty of Homoeopathy,
Royal London Homoeopathic
Hospital, Great Ormond Street,
London WC1N 3HR
Tel: 020 7837 3091

Homoeopathic Hospital,
1000 Great Western Road,
Glasgow G12 0NR
Tel: 0141 339 0382

The British Homoeopathic Association,
27a Devonshire Street, London
WC1N 1RJ
Tel: 020 7935 2163
Fax: 020 7486 2957
Website:www.nhsconfed.net/bha

Homoeopathic Trust Faculty of Homoeopathy,
Hahnemann House, 2 Powis
Place, London WC1N 3HT
Tel: 020 7837 9469

The Society of Homoeopaths,
2 Artisan Road, Northampton
NN1 4HU
Tel: 01604 621400
Fax: 01604 622622
Email: societyofhomoeopaths@
btinternet.com
Website:
www.homoeopathy.org.uk

Hypnotherapy

British Society of Medical and Dental Hypnotists,
73 Ware Street, Hertford
SG13 7ED
Tel: 020 8905 4342

British Hypnotherapy Association,
67 Upper Berkeley Street,
London W1
Tel: 020 7723 4443

National Council of Hypnotherapy,
Hazelwood, Broadmead,
Lymington, Hampshire
SO41 6DH

Central Register of Advanced Hypnotherapists (CRAH),
28 Finsbury Park Road,
London N4 2JX
Tel: 020 7359 6991

Iridology

Guild of Naturopathic Iridologists,
94 Grosvenor Road, London
SW1V 3LF
Tel/fax: 020 7821 0255
Website:
www.gni-inter national.org

Jin Shin Jyutsu

Southsea Centre for Complementary Medicine,
25 Osborne Road, Southsea,
Hants PO5 3ND
Tel: 01705 874748

Kinesiology

Association of Systematic Kinesiology,
39 Browns Road, Surbiton,
Surrey KT5 8ST
Tel: 020 8399 3215
Fax: 020 8390 1010
Email: info@kinesiology.co.uk
Website: www.kinesiology.co.uk

Kinesiology Federation,
PO Box 7891, Wimbledon,
London SW19 1ZB
Tel: 020 8545 0255

Massage

Clare Maxwell Hudson School of Massage,
PO Box 457, London NW2 4BR
Tel: 020 8450 6494
Website:
www.cmhmassage.co.uk

Massage Therapy Institute of Great Britain,
PO Box 2726, London NW2 4NR
Tel: 020 8208 1607
Fax: 020 8208 1639
(national register of practitioners)

London College of Massage,
5 Newman Passage, London
W1P 3P
Tel: 020 7323 3574
Fax: 020 7637 7125

Meditation

London Zen Society,
10 Belmont Street, London NW1
Tel: 020 7485 9576

London Soto Zen Group,
23 Westbere Road, London NW2
Tel: 020 7794 3109

Transcendental Meditation UK,
Beacon House, Willow Walk,
Woodley Park, Skelmersdale,
Lancs WN8 6UR
Tel: 08705 143733
(for your nearest TM centre)
Email: info@transcendental-
meditation.org.uk
Website: www.transcendental-
meditation.org.uk

Naturopathy

General Council and Register of Naturopaths & Naturopathic Helpline,
Goswell House, 2 Goswell Road,
Street, Somerset BA16 0JG
Tel: 01458 840072

Incorporated Society of British Naturopaths,
The Coach House,
293 Gilmerton Road, Edinburgh
EH16 5UQ
Tel: 0131 664 3435

Nutritional Therapy

Society for the Promotion of Nutritional Therapy,
PO Box 85, St Albans,
Herts AL3 72Q
Tel: 01582 792088
Email: spnt@compuserve.com
Website:
www.visitweb.com/spnt

Osteopathy

British Osteopathic Association,
Langham House East, Mill Street,
Bedfordshire LU1 2NA
Tel: 01582 488455

The Osteopathic Information Centre,
Room 432, Premier House,
10 Greycoat Place, London
SW1P 13B
Tel: 020 7799 2442

Pilates

Body Control Suite,
17 Queensberry Mews West,
London SW7 2DY
Tel: 020 7581 7041
Fax: 020 7581 2286
Website:
www.bodycontrol.co.uk

The Balanced Body Studios,
150 Chiswick High Road,
Chiswick, London W4 1PR
Tel: 020 8742 8311
Email: enquiry@pilates.uk.com

Polarity

UK Polarity Therapy Association,
Monomark House, 27 Old
Gloucester Street, London
WC1N 3XX
Tel: 01483 417714
Email: ukpta@avnet.co.uk

International School of Polarity Therapy,
12-14 Dowell Street, Honiton,
Devon EX14 8LT
Tel: 01404 44330

Reflexology

The British School of Reflexology,
Holistic Healing Centre, 92
Sheering Road, Old Harlow,
Essex CM17 0JW
Tel: 01279 429060
Fax: 01279 445234

The British Reflexology Association,
Monks Orchard, Whitbourne,
Worcester WR6 5RB
Tel: 01886 821207
Fax: 01886 822017
Email: bra@britreflex.co.uk
Website: www.britreflex.co.uk

Metamorphic Association,
New Cross Therapy Centre,
67 Ritherdon Road, Balham,
London SW17 8QE
Tel: 020 8672 5951
Email: metamorphic@
britishisles.freeserve.co.uk

Reiki

International Reiki Society,
PO Box 1867, Yeovil, Somerset
BA22 7YU
Tel: 0797 0357362

Reiki Association,
2 Manor Cottages, Stockley Hill,
Peterchurch, Hereford HR2 0SS
Tel: 01981 550829

Rolfing

Rolf Institute,
80 Clifton Hill, London NW8 0JT
Tel: 020 7328 90268

Shiatsu

The Shiatsu Society,
31 Pullman Lane, Godalming,
Surrey GU7 1XY
Tel: 01483 860771

Sound Therapy

Association of Professional Music Therapists,
38 Pierce Lane, Fulbourne,
Cambridge CB1 5BL
Tel: 01223 880377

T'ai Chi Ch'uan

British T'ai Chi Ch'uan Association,
7 Upper Wimpole Street,
London W1M 7TD
Tel: 020 7935 8444

The T'ai Chi Union for Great Britain,
94 Felsham Road,
London SW15 1DQ
Tel: 020 8780 1063
Email: cromptonph@aol.com

Yoga

British Wheel of Yoga,
1 Hamilton Place, Boston Road,
Sleaford, Lincolnshire NG34 7ES
Tel: 01529 306851
Fax: 01529 303233

Yoga Biomedical Trust,
The Royal London
Homoeopathic Hospital
(see General addresses)
Tel: 020 7419 7195
Fax: 020 7419 7196
Email: yogabio.med@virgin.net
Website: www.yogatherapy.org
(Special classes for pregnancy
and postnatal groups)

The Yoga for Health Foundation,
Ickwell Bury, Ickwell Green,
Bedfordshire SG18 9EF
Tel: 01767 627271
Fax: 01767 627266

Zero Balancing

Zero Balance Association UK,
10 Victoria Grove, Bridport
DT6 3AA
Tel: 01308 420097

AUSTRALIA

Australian Natural Therapists Association,
PO Box 308, Melrose Park,
South Australia 5039
Tel: 08 297 9533
Fax: 08 297 0003

Australian Traditional Medicine Society,
PO Box 442, Suite 3, First Floor,
120 Blaxland Road, Ryde,
NSW 2122
Tel: 02 808 2825
Fax: 02 809 7570

Australian Women's Health Network,
PO Box 400, Dickson, ACT 2609
Tel: 03 5444 7569 *or*
03 9777 0541
Fax: 03 5444 7977
Website: www.awhn.org.au

Nursing Mothers' Association of Australia,
5 Glendale Street, PO Box 231,
Nunawading, Victoria 3131
Tel: 03 9877 2211
Fax: 03 9695 0790

Australian Council on Chiropractic and Osteopathic Education,
941 Nepean Highway,
Mornington, Victoria 3931

Australian Institute of Homeopathy,
21 Bulah Close, Berdwara
Heights, NSW 2082

Australasian College of Natural Therapies,
57 Foveaux Street, Surry Hills,
NSW 2010
Tel: 02 9218 88500
Fax: 02 9281 4411
E-mail: info@acnt.edu.au

The Childbirth Education Association of Australia (NSW),
PO Box 413, Hurstville BC,
NSW 1481
Tel: 9580 0399
Fax: 9580 9986
Website: www.cea-nsw.com.au

NEW ZEALAND

Canterbury College of Natural Medicine,
PO Box 4329, Christchurch
Tel: 03 366 0373
Fax: 03 366 5342

New Zealand Natural Health Practitioners Accreditation Board,
PO Box 37-491, Auckland
Tel: 09 625 9966

New Zealand Homoeopathic Society,
PO Box 67095, Mount Eden,
Auckland
Tel:

New Zealand Register of Acupuncturists,
PO Box 9950, Wellington 1
Tel/Fax: 04 476 8578

SOUTH AFRICA

The Centre for Natural Therapies and the School of Complementary Health,
475 Townbush Road, Montrose,
Pietermaritzburg 3201 *or*
PO Box 13559, Cascades 3202
Tel: 033 347 3937
Fax: 033 347 0680

Nutrition Information Centre,
Nicus, PO Box 19063,
Tygerberg 7505
Tel: 021 933 1408
Fax: 021 933 1405

South Africa Homoeopaths, Chiropractors and Allied Professions Board,
PO Box 17055, 0027 Groenkloof
Tel: 246 6455

USA

American Holistic Association,
4101 Lake Boone Trail, Suite 201,
Raleigh, NC 27607
Tel: 919 787 5181

National Association of Childbearing Centres,
3123 Gottschall Road, 1518
Perkiomenville, PA 18074
Tel: 215 234 8068

National Women's Health Network,
514 10th Street NW,
Washington, DC 20037
Tel: 202 347 1140

Office of Alternative Medicine Information Center,
National Institute of Health, Suite
405, 6120 Executive Blvd,
Rockville, MD 20892-9904
Tel: 301 402 2466

Society for Nutrition Education,
2001 Kilebrew Drive, Suite 340,
Minneapolis, MN 55425
Tel: 612 854 0035

American Association of Acupuncture and Oriental Medicine,
4101 Lake Boone Trail, Suite 210,
Raleigh, NC 27607
Tel: 919 787 5181

American Society of Teachers of the Alexander Technique,
PO Box 517, Urbana,
IL 61801-0517
Tel: 080 473 0620
Website: www.alexandertech.org

American Aromatherapy Association,
PO Box 3679, South Pasadena,
CA 91031
Tel: 818 457 1742

American Institute of Vedic Studies,
PO Box 8357, Santa Fe,
NM 87501
Tel: 505 983 9385
(Correspondence course)

Dr Edward Bach Healing Society,
644 Merrick Road, Lynbrook,
NY 11563
Tel: 516 593 2206

American Chiropractic Association,
1701 Clarendon Blvd, Arlington,
VA 22209
Tel: 703 276 8800
Website: www.amerchiro.org

Hellerwork International,
406 Berry Street, Mount Shasta,
CA 96067
Tel: 916 926 2500

American Herbalists Guild,
PO Box 70, Roosevelt, UT 84066
Tel: 435 722 8434
Fax: 435 722 8452
Email: ahgoffice@earthlink.net

National Centre for Homoeopathy,
801 North Fairfax Street,
Alexandria, VA 22314
Tel: 703 548 7790

American Society of Clinical Hypnosis,
2200 East Devon Avenue,
Des Plaines, IL 60018
Tel: 847 297 3317

The Jin Shen Do Foundation,
PO Box 1097, Felton, CA 95018
Tel: 408 338 9454

International College of Applied Kinesiology,
PO Box 905, Lawrence,
KA 66044 0905
Tel: 913 542 1801

American Massage Therapy Association,
820 Davis Street, Evanston,
IL 60201
Tel: 708 864 0123
Website: www.amtamassage.org

American Association of Naturopathic Physicians,
2366 Eastlake Ave East, Seattle,
WA 98102
Tel: 206 323 7610

American Osteopathic Association,
142 East Ontario Street, Chicago,
IL 60611
Tel: 312 280 5800

The Pilates Info Homepage
Website: www.hermit.
com/hermit.org.htm
(For a full list of American teachers and studios)

The Polarity Therapy Center of San Francisco,
409-A Lawton Street,
San Francisco, CA 94122
Tel: 415 753 1298

International Institute of Reflexology,
PO Box 12642, St Petersburg,
FL 33733
Tel: 813 343 4811

Centre for Reiki Healing,
29209 Northwestern Highway
593, Southfield, MI 48034-9841

Rolf Institute,
205 Canyon Boulevard, Boulder,
CO 80302
Tel: 303 449 5903

Touch for Health Foundation,
1174 North Lake Avenue,
Pasadena, CA 91104-3797
Tel: 818 794 1181

International Association of Yoga Therapists,
109 Hillside Ave, Mill Valley,
CA 94941
Tel: 415 383 4587

INDEX